A TIME TO FIGHT

Second Edition

This book is dedicated to God who gives us strength,

To Morgan and Dylan, our brave and strong kids,

To Linda and Jack Park, our parents who took care of us,

To Dr. Fredrick Hagemeister, the world's greatest lymphoma doctor,

And to cancer patients and caregivers all around the world - you're our heroes.

It was a cold, dark October morning. We had not come prepared for the 40-degree temperature and cool winds. The three of us sat on the small hill overlooking the lake, wrapped in a tiny blanket, awaiting the start of the race. Shivering, we watched as race officials and volunteers laid out orange cones and set up the finish line. None of us had ever been to a triathlon event and although we were thrilled to be there, we were miserable waiting.

An hour later, we heard the emcee announce there was a special racer there that day. "Lets all hear it for Bill Crews," he said, "who finished chemotherapy five months ago and is competing in his first triathlon today." My two children looked up at me with glowing, proud eyes. "They're talking about Daddy," they screamed. I smiled and felt a new warmth. Soon the sun began to rise and sparkle like tiny stars upon the lake. Body-marked and transition set up, triathletes began to walk about and some of the very brave ones even jumped into the lake to get a little swim in. Then I saw Bill. Nervous and happy, he walked over and hugged us. We talked for a few moments before he was off again. "Good luck," we all smiled. We had no idea what kinds of emotion this day would bring and what an amazing victory our family was claiming in those few short hours that beautiful October morning.

Exactly one year earlier, life as we'd known it, was forever changed. Without warning, a cruel enemy flooded our world and shattered our home. The four of us, bound together by love and God's strength, fought for our lives and took that enemy down. This is our story...

THE FIGHT BEGINS

To everything there is a season, A time for every purpose under heaven...

Dana-Susan

October 14, 2003 was a humid Houston morning. Although it was Tuesday, my children were not at school. They attended a private preschool and kindergarten where I was the Spanish teacher. We only attended school three days each week, so Tuesdays were usually set aside to have play dates and practice swimming. This morning was a little different. My husband Bill, who had turned 37 years old the month before, kissed me goodbye that morning and headed to his orthopedic doctor to get the results of an MRI done on his shoulder. He'd been experiencing great pain for a few weeks and eventually wasn't able to move either of his arms. Because we were swimmers, we figured he'd torn his rotator cuff and might need surgery. His doctor felt certain that was the case as well. Bill was especially anxious about it because he had been training with the idea in mind of doing a triathlon. As a swimmer, he had achieved as many of his goals as he had desired. It was time for a newer, bigger challenge. He'd put in the hours of running, cycling, swimming and weightlifting and was growing more and more excited to branch out into the world of multisport.

Although I thought it a little exciting for Bill, I wasn't too terribly interested in triathlon. Actually, the idea of getting back into competitive sports seemed crazy to me. We were too busy. Besides careers and children, we were very involved in extracurricular activities as well. We volunteered coaching swimming and soccer. We participated in Habitat for Humanity and many other charities. Our fitness program was already fulfilling enough. I was doing Pilates, swimming, kickboxing and weightlifting while Bill trained hard every day on his own. Our children were becoming very strong little swimmers and soccer players. Life was certainly busy. And it was very good. I actually sat thinking about how lucky we were that day. We were strong and healthy and active. All we needed now was for Bill to get this problem with his shoulder taken care of so we could get back out there.

It had all happened so quickly. Days following his birthday, we were outside talking to our neighbor about the big race I was participating in with Habitat for Humanity. It was a day filled with rowing and other sports and the entire community was involved. This was normally an event Bill loved to participate in for his company, but his shoulder had been hurting and he was thinking of going to the doctor. This year, I would compete and he would be my cheerleader. A couple of days after the sports event, Bill went for a swim. After he swam laps, his shoulder was in so much pain, he could barely move it. Although he didn't know it at the time, that would be his last swim for many months. By the next morning, the pain was so intense, he could not move either arm. Soon, his chest was hurting too. He called his doctor and scheduled an appointment for two days later, a Thursday morning.

That morning, I left with the kids and got my class started for the day. An hour later, I decided to call and check on Bill and make sure he was up and getting to his appointment. There was such a dark feeling in the air. I couldn't quite comprehend it. Part of it was the fact that half of my students had become suddenly ill and were sent home with fever. Part of it was the approaching thunderstorm. Bill's voice was so weak and when I asked how he was doing, he told me how he'd been unable to remove his shirt to take a shower and had cut it off his body with scissors. "If you're having that much trouble moving your arms, I think I'll come home and drive you to the doctor," I said. My boss told me to leave and not to worry about my students. A substitute was on her way to my class.

When I walked through the door of our home, the storm hit. I grabbed the umbrella and found Bill lying on the bed, barely able to move. "My chest hurts," he said quietly. It was still too early for us to go to the doctor, but I was frightened. "What if he's having a heart attack", I thought. I drove through torrential rains only to find that the clinic was closed for lunch. A receptionist told us that if his chest was hurting, we should get him to the emergency room. So I drove back through the harsh winds and rain, about a 30-minute drive and checked Bill in at the emergency room. The wait wasn't too bad, but I began to wonder if we'd make it back in time to pick up our children from school. I phoned a friend who would pick them up and take them to my neighbor's house. That settled, I was able to concentrate on my husband. He didn't seem right. I had seen him suffer through intense migraines for many years. He had endured great suffering in his life, including various surgeries and nearly losing his life when a horse kicked him in his kidney, forcing him to spend a month in the ICU. He knew how to handle pain, yet something about this day seemed dismal.

Once they called his name and asked all the questions, it seemed they were going to quickly rule out a heart attack. That was good. Still, something was wrong and I couldn't believe it was only a torn rotator cuff. He just seemed to be in too much pain. The doctor came in later and told us to go home and keep our appointment with the orthopedic doctor. "I truly believe it's a torn rotator cuff," he said, "and those can hurt pretty bad."

We left that evening with no real answers, but I was relieved. Things could have been worse, I told myself. At least it's not his heart and if he needs surgery, well, he can get through that. I accompanied my husband to his orthopedic doctor's visit. He could not drive. An X-ray revealed very little, so an MRI was ordered for that night. Bill received a Cortisone shot to help ease the pain and we left.

Because he wasn't hurting nearly as bad after the shot, Bill was able to drive himself to the MRI building that night. It was a Friday night so we knew we'd have to be patient and wait maybe several days for results. Meanwhile, we were glad for the pain relief and hopeful that a surgery date would be set quickly so he could get through physical therapy and get back to training for that triathlon.

What a surprise when we didn't have to wait that long for results after all. By Monday afternoon, the doctor phoned and told Bill he wanted to see him first thing in the morning. Things were happening fast.

Not long after he left, I was surprised to hear from him so

quickly. When I answered the phone, I hoped the surgery was already set and he would be able to get his shoulder back to functioning in no time. Immediately I heard the fear in his trembling voice. "They think it's cancer," Bill quietly said.

My very first thought was, "there must be a mistake" followed instantly by "we're going to fight hard against this." While I waited for him to return, I got on the phone and called my parents who had just flown in from their home in Europe two days before. I couldn't believe the sound of the words coming out of my mouth as I told my mom my husband had cancer. "This can't be," I said, "it's not what God has planned for Bill." As soon as I said that, it hit me that maybe this was exactly the plan. It might just be that this was God's way of placing us exactly where He'd always intended for us to be. She and I only talked for a couple of minutes before I hung up to call our church and ask if we could stop by and pray with the pastor. Before we knew anything at all about the battle ahead, I knew we had better start the fight the right way. Our first weapon would be prayer.

It was a 15-minute drive home for Bill and one of the greatest regrets of my life was that I was not with him when the doctor gave him the news. He had faced it alone and was now driving alone, facing all kinds of uncertainties. Cancer was such an ugly word to him. When he was only eight years old his six-year-old sister Michelle died of leukemia. He'd felt great pain at such an early age. Cancer was not only a terrible disease, but also a thief, robbing him of a little sister he loved dearly and stealing his family's joy. While I waited, I prepared myself to be his strength and confidence, his rock to stand on. I was determined not to cry or be afraid, but to remain calm. It's what he had always done for me, so I figured I owed him.

Bill

As I walked from the doctor's office to my Jeep with the MRI slides under my arm, I wondered how I was going to call and break the news to my young wife. All I'd ever known of cancer was that it killed people. It had killed my sister, both of my grandfathers, and some very good friends. I'd never personally known anyone who had survived cancer. I felt like I might have just been given a death sentence and wondered how much longer I had and what kind of torture I was facing. I waited until I got to the highway before I called Dana-Susan. This was one of the hardest phone calls I ever had to make. How would she react? Would hearing her voice make me lose it?

When she answered the phone, I could hardly get the words out because I started tearing up immediately. I was actually about to say those words out loud for the first time. Hearing myself say I had cancer was strange. Dana-Susan seemed shocked, but strong. "What," she quickly responded.

"They think it's cancer," I repeated, "and I'm going to MD Anderson Thursday." I tried to briefly explain the results of the MRI. I did not have a torn rotator cuff. My shoulder bone was apparently dead and my bone marrow had abnormalities that looked like maybe leukemia. *Leukemia*. Now that was the ugliest word I'd ever heard.

My 31-year-old friend had just died of leukemia only a few months before. My sister died of leukemia many years before. I loathe that disease. Was it possible that I might have it? Or was it bone cancer? My doctor didn't know. He only knew that I needed to get into the cancer center as soon as possible. The urgency of it all made this drive home all the more excruciating. Dana-Susan suddenly seemed very calm and very confident, like she knew exactly what to do and nothing was going to keep her from doing it. I knew she would call her parents to get them to start praying. I didn't know what she planned for after that. She was pretty resolute. I hung up and desperately wanted to get home. It seemed like it took forever to get there. I cried all the way.

Dana-Susan

Bill came home from his appointment and we went immediately to church where the pastor prayed with us. We knew he would pray with passion because he knows the devastation of cancer. His sister died of leukemia in 1990. That kind of loss is so great it cannot be measured.

When we left church that day, I felt two things hit at once. The first was peace. It was hard to comprehend, but I had peace that no matter what we were facing, God would be on our side. The second was that a definite war had begun. How could it be possible to feel peace and war all at once? But that's what I felt – a surge of peace and the spirit of war rise inside me. I knew we were only beginning the fight.

A time to laugh...

Dana-Susan

When Bill and I met, I was impressed by his cheerfulness and love for life. He was energetic and fun, and we became instant friends. We shared many common interests and hobbies, most especially physical fitness. We swam competitively and Bill even volunteered as a swim coach for the Texas Amateur Athletic Federation. On June 1, 1996, we got married. A storm blew through Dallas. Some people were unable to drive through the streets. Rains and wind were worse than we'd seen them in a very long time. I knew the storms were raging outside, but there I was in the bridal suite smiling. I was at peace. In only a short while, I would be clinging to my daddy's arm as he slowly walked me down the aisle to marry my best friend. So I had a sure calm in the midst of a vicious storm. The minister used that cruel weather to make some very valid points about marriage and life. "The storms of life will hit," he said, but he said Bill and I would survive those storms together. I believed that. When the reception was over early that evening and we were ready to leave, the storms ceased. Deep blue Texas sky and a warm, gentle breeze were our send-off as our guests kissed us and waved goodbye.

We honeymooned at a Mexican beach resort. Most of the days were bright and sunny, but one evening a huge storm blew through the city. We sat at the outdoor bar watching as the sea screamed violently. Barstools and umbrellas flew through the dark air. We watched in amazement, and I found it almost amusing that our wedding and honeymoon had both been victims of brutal storms. I thought about the "storms of life" we'd been warned about days before. And I thought about how Bill and I were calmly sitting together unafraid. We didn't cower to the storm, retreating to our room to seek shelter. We enjoyed ourselves together, laughing in the midst of the fierce winds, lightning and thunder.

Life presented us with many storms, but we safely made it through them all. Through every trial, our faith was deepened, and a bond of unity built between us. In the first two years of our marriage, we worked together with the swim team, traveled and enjoyed our youth. We loved our life. And then it got even better. We had our first child. She was perfect – a sweet, pretty girl with bright blue eyes. Morgan was a great delight. When she was born, I was still teaching junior high school in a Dallas suburb and Bill was in the oil and gas industry. Four months later, we were being transferred to Houston. We moved into a lovely suburb north of the city called The Woodlands. It was ideal for us, fitting our personality and lifestyle. Snug in the forested area, this master-planned community had miles of trails, parks and vast outdoor activity. We felt very at home. Soon we were having our second child, our son Dylan. He and Morgan made our lives complete.

It was while I was pregnant with Dylan that I'd get a foretaste of battling suffering and pain. We were practicing diving at the Woodlands Athletic Center. Morgan was an exceptional diver for a 23-month-old. But I watched closely each time she climbed that metal ladder and held her hand from down below as she walked out to the end of the diving board. Bill waited in the water for her to dive in, make a splash, and then swim toward him. On about the 20th dive of the night, I called, "last one" and little Morgan slowly climbed up the ladder. This time, though, her foot got caught and slipped through the bars. In a second, I saw my tiny little girl fall from the one-meter diving board, head first into the cement pool deck. That was the longest couple of seconds of my life as I ran to her, picked her up in my arms and suddenly heard her scream. Moments later, as she vomited violently, we were racing to the emergency room to find out she'd fractured her skull. For years following that night, I played it over and over again in my mind. I was the mom. I should have never allowed that to happen to my baby. What kind of horrible mother does that? For many months following, Morgan suffered headaches and high fevers and although the doctors told me none of it related to the fall, I constantly blamed myself. Eventually we would learn the truth that she is, unfortunately, a migraine sufferer.

I don't always understand why we suffer, but I have learned that suffering is such a great way to build character and develop patience. During the time of difficulty, it's not fun, but later, after it has built strength and endurance, it's worth it. Morgan has learned a great deal about endurance and overcoming trouble by some of the pain in her young life. When her brother came along, it was obvious he too would learn those valuable life lessons at an early age.

Dylan smiled the day he was born. Some people think it's not possible. No, it's just a reflex, they say. As his mother, I disagree.

He smiled and he meant to smile. He smiled every day after he was born too. If I made a funny face, he would smile. If I sang a song, he smiled. I think Dylan was just a happy guy. He was 30 days old when our friend Debby was in town staying with us. She sat with me as I got him ready for bed and fed him for the last time of the night. "He's so happy," she remarked. Several hours later, as we all slept, Dylan began to cry. I picked him up, thinking it was time for him to eat again and was shocked to feel his tiny body. I checked his temperature, and his fever was more than 103 degrees. Bill got on the phone with the doctor who said to take him immediately to the emergency room. They told us they were not trained to handle infants, but tried to do a spinal tap anyway. It didn't work so they tried again. And again. I was quickly losing patience, but trying to hold back my feelings. Then they called for the ambulance and sent my baby boy to Texas Children's Hospital in Houston. I had no idea what was wrong and once again found myself fretting for my child's life.

They did three more spinal taps unsuccessfully because the damage had already been done at the other hospital. Dylan was admitted to the hospital with high fever, and we were forced to just hope it was nothing too serious. My mom and dad accompanied us to the hospital. As we walked through those halls my dad reminisced. He'd had his share of dad duty in those halls. For him and my mom, their memories probably seemed not so far in the past. For me, those dark days of life at Texas Children's Hospital many years ago came darting back again too. It was a different era and a different fight, but a fight our family will never forget.

Day after day I stayed in Dylan's room. I only left once to go down to the lobby and visit Morgan who had been staying with my mom. I was only four weeks postpartum and feeling very ill myself. Often, I would wonder why my side hurt so badly, but figured it must be the stress on top of the fact that I'd just delivered a big baby boy. For seven days, we stayed in that place and then finally the fever dropped enough to send him home. I guess we'll never know for sure, but for some reason, the doctor there felt that Dylan's immune system was deficient. At any rate, he got better, and we went home. I, on the other hand, did not get better. My side hurt pretty badly. But I told Bill I was fine and he could go. He was working in Fort Worth for a few months, coming home only on the weekends. It wasn't easy having an infant and a toddler and being on my own. I figured this pain would go away over time if I got some rest. But I was wrong.

One very early morning a few days later, I fell to the floor in Dylan's room. It was 4:00 a.m. and I couldn't think of anyone to phone at such an unreasonable hour. I waited until 7:00 and then called my mom. I told her about my pain and she told me I needed to go to the emergency room. I was beginning to think of that place as my second home. My brother came to help with the kids while my mom accompanied me to the hospital. A few hours later, I was being prepped for surgery to remove my appendix which was about to rupture. Bill caught a plane and made it just in time to kiss me before I was asleep.

After surgery, I was tired. I'd just delivered a baby and spent a week with him in the hospital and then had surgery. I wasn't sure if I was really strong enough to deal with it all. Strength, I began to learn, is built over time and through adversity. So maybe I wasn't strong at first, but I was getting stronger every day.

Eventually life got settled down. Morgan and Dylan were healthy, happy children and Bill was no longer in Fort Worth. The storms of life calmed a little and we enjoyed a time of great joy and laughter. Or maybe it was just the calm before another devastating storm.

A time to mourn...

Bill

*A*s a young boy, I always enjoyed my summers. When school was out I would get to spend time in central Texas with my family. We often made trips to Salado, a small country town, to visit my uncle and aunt's ranch. My dad's whole side of the family lived near there, most of them on big ranches or farms. My sister, Michelle, and I used to love to chase chickens around the farm or go fishing with my parents.

During these vacations, we stayed at my grandparents' house in Killeen. My parents and baby brother Jamie slept in a room at the back of the house we called the "den" while Michelle and I slept on day beds in a tiny room with red carpets we called "the little room".

The last weekend in May 1974, we made one of our family trips to central Texas. Early that Saturday morning, we congregated in the living room of my grandparents' house getting ready for a fishing trip to Salado. My grandmother commented that Michelle looked a little pale, but nothing more was made of it. Soon, we piled into two cars and headed to one of my cousin's ranches in Salado. It was a short drive and before long, we were at the pond doing what we loved most.

While my dad and I fished, my mom took Michelle and Jamie to the house to go to the bathroom. Moments later, she screamed for my dad. He and I rushed to find my sister passed out beside my mom on the hillside.

My next memory is of my parents driving away with my sister to the hospital while Jamie and I got into my grandparents' car to head back to their house. I walked into the house and into the "little room" and asked "Is Michelle going to die?" Then I sat on one of the day beds and broke into tears. I don't know why my mind went right away to the thought of death.

Michelle spent the next several days in Scott and White Hospital in Temple, Texas as the doctors tried to find out what was wrong with her. I spent that time at my grandparents' house frightened and feeling very alone. Later my family would tell me that my five-year-old sister had something called leukemia. As a seven-year-old boy, that was a totally foreign word to me. My little sister and I had been best friends. We played games together and loved swimming. Michelle was a happy, friendly little girl who loved people and laughter. From the moment they drove away with her, it seemed that laughter went too.

Once we returned to our home in Dallas, our lives became regular visits to Children's Hospital. Although I don't remember every visit, I do remember certain things. I remember there always being many people in the leukemia area. I remember all the other kids with leukemia and how sick they were. I remember how obvious it was when some of the kids would disappear from one visit to the next. Leukemia took most children's lives back then. You never knew who would be the next to go. Michelle would usually have to get her finger pricked for blood work. She said it hurt pretty badly, but after it was over, she was given a finger puppet to put over her finger with the bandage. We collected enough of those finger puppets between May and December that we were able to use them alone to decorate our Christmas tree.

One hospital visit that really stands out in my mind was a trip to the radiation area. We had to stay outside of the room that Michelle was in. We watched her on a monitor as she was put through a big donut-shaped machine. It all seemed so scary. The radiation and chemotherapy she went through caused her to lose her hair. Most of the time, she wore a wig, but she couldn't wear it when she went swimming. As a big brother, I was protective of Michelle so it made me very angry when kids would make fun of her at the pool.

Life the year of Michelle's sickness was hard on me and my family, but even harder was her death. One year after her diagnosis, in May 1975, I was taking some of the classroom books back to the storage closet in our school when the secretary asked me how Michelle was doing. I told her what I had been told. Michelle was in the hospital with chicken pox, but she was getting better and would be coming home soon. I left school that day, the last day of second grade, and went home with a smile. It seemed like our troubles were finally over.

I was not prepared for what I heard as I walked through the front door of my house. My grandmother looked into my eyes and simply said, "Your sister died today." Suddenly, without warning, nothing would ever be the same again.

I don't remember the next few days. I don't remember talking to my parents. My only vivid memory following that last day of school is of our family walking sadly into the funeral home. I remember leaning over the coffin to see my sister lying motionless. I leaned closer to kiss her cheek and felt how cold and lifeless it was. Cancer had stolen my sister and changed my life forever.

Dana-Susan

It always seemed at least a little interesting to me that Bill and I both know what it's like to be a child with a very ill sibling. We both experienced the leukemia section of a children's hospital early in life and it has impacted our outlook on life. When I was seven years old, my baby brother Luke was diagnosed with a very rare pediatric cancer known as langerhans cell histiocytosis. He was only 18 months old and was facing an almost certain death as doctors at Texas Children's Hospital explained that no one under the age of three had ever acquired this disease to this extent and survived. Because the disease behaves like a combination of both blood and bone cancer, young patients are treated with chemotherapy and radiation. The disease is caused by an excess of white blood cells that cluster together and attack the skin, bones, lung, liver, spleen, gums, ears, eyes and the central nervous system. In my brother's case, the X-rays of his skull and spine looked like Swiss cheese as his bones were being eaten away.

Luke endured the torment and pain of other young patients with blood cancer and bone cancer as he stayed in the leukemia section. I remember seeing all those bald, dying children and

21

thinking how wrong it seemed. Kids are supposed to be outdoors, running and laughing, not shut up inside a cold, sterile hospital doing chemotherapy and radiation. Luke was brave, filled with courage even as a baby. He suffered through bone marrow aspirations and biopsies of his brain. He patiently withstood chemotherapy and even smiled through his pain. I learned a lot from my brother.

I also learned a lot from my parents. They were the epitome of faithfulness. They never wavered in their trust in God. It wasn't until they walked through the halls of Texas Children's Hospital years later with Dylan and me that I was finally able to slightly comprehend what that battle was like for them. Their tiny baby was doing chemo and doctors were telling them he would die.

When all the odds were against him, Luke survived. He wasn't supposed to live and if he did, he certainly wasn't supposed to live well. But he defied his disease and went on to live a very healthy, normal life. Our family's faith in God increased during that trying time. We also learned how to stand together against a common enemy. Although I didn't know it at the time, this was a foretaste of another family I would someday have, standing together against a common enemy.

When Bill and I first got married, we wondered if there was some plan or purpose for us in helping families dealing with cancer. We'd both seen the darkness and fear of cancer from an early age. It had done something to us as individuals, making our hearts tender toward families with cancer. Now we wondered if as a couple we could do anything to help.

Years later, our friend Chad died of leukemia in January 2003. Chad was a wonderful young man filled with life. His death was tragic for his sweet young wife and two precious children. His parents and his friends and family were grieved.

A couple of months later while we visited with my parents in their home in Spain, Bill and I told them about our desire to do something to somehow help families dealing with cancer. They loved the idea and encouraged us to pursue it. On the way home, I sat on the plane and had a very strong feeling that very soon we would be heading to MD Anderson Cancer Center in Houston. I was right.

A time to weep...

Dana-Susan

Two days after the results of the MRI had shocked us, Bill and I made our first visit down to The University of Texas MD Anderson Cancer Center in the heart of the medical center in Houston, Texas. As we stepped out of the car and handed our keys to the valet, Bill grabbed his folder with MRI results and we walked through the big, glass doors. This place was massive. We walked slowly to the desk marked "New Patient Registration". I felt like we were in the lobby of a big hotel. Bill signed in and we found a couch to sit on and began our first of many long waits. Moments later I excused myself to go to the ladies' room.

I was feeling queasy. All of this was very overwhelming. When I walked into the restroom, I heard someone vomiting. I cringed. A tall, thin, bald-headed woman walked out, wiped her face and washed her hands so very matter-of-factly. I walked into the stall, looked up to Heaven and said, "God I know this must be a mistake because I can't handle this." Some people think God doesn't give us things we can't handle. I'm not so sure. He has given me lots of things I can't handle, but I think He handles a lot of it for me.

I returned to the couch to sit next to my anxious husband. I took a quick glance at him sitting there. He was so strong and healthy. All his life he'd been an exceptional athlete, winning many medals and trophies in swimming and soccer. He had even been a bull rider. For years he'd been in top physical condition, cross-training and weightlifting. His body was rock solid. It was quite difficult to believe he could actually have cancer in that tough, fit body.

Bill

I sat there in the midst of this busy place filled with the commotion of cancer patients walking to and from their appointments, volunteers pushing coffee carts and the many others sitting, waiting. We did a lot of waiting in those days. I kept hoping there had been a mistake and that unlike all these others sitting in the lobby with their MRI's, I would be sent home and told I didn't have cancer after all.

Dana-Susan

Soon, a kind woman walked out and called, "William Crews, Jr.". We got up and followed her to a tiny office where mountains of papers filled the desk. She began to interview Bill about his insurance policy and he sat filling out more paperwork. It all began to feel so real. When she was finished, she handed him a blue card with his patient identification. It was official. In front of my eyes, the athlete became the cancer patient.

Next, we walked to the elevator and headed up to the orthopedic center. Still not knowing what kind of cancer we were facing, we clung to hope that it was something simple and easy to cure. We began another very long wait while Bill filled out even more papers. This time, they were all about his health. One question after another caused me to wonder why we were here. Bill seemed almost relieved as he began to check "no" to all the symptoms. Had I not been there he definitely would have checked "no" on them all. "Do you have night sweats," one question read. As he began to check "no", I stopped him. What was he thinking? "Every night I threaten to stop sleeping in the same bed with you because of all that nasty sweating", I thought. "Do you itch?" Weird question, we agreed, but he had to check "yes" because for months I had been irritated at his constant scratching.

When the nurse finally called for him, we rose with the papers and waited for a while in the exam room. Then the nurse began interviewing him, asking the same questions he'd already answered on the papers. Bill seemed almost too hyper to me. I could tell he desperately wanted this all to be a mistake, so he seemed too happy when he could say he didn't have most of the symptoms listed.

Within half an hour, a doctor who was a fellow entered the room. MD Anderson is a teaching hospital and often the fellows will examine the patients before the main doctor comes in. This young doctor asked many of the same questions as before while he examined Bill. I watched closely. Then he asked, "How long have you had this lump?"

Stunned, I looked up and saw a large lump in Bill's armpit. "Oh that," Bill answered calmly, "I noticed it a couple of months ago. I think it's just a damaged muscle from my weight training program."

The doctor coolly said, "We'll need to get a biopsy". Moments later, the main doctor entered. A tall, good-looking orthopedic doctor, he smiled and shook our hands. He carried in the MRI results we'd brought with us that day and hung them up to the light. He and the fellow talked to each other about the lump while I shot Bill a look of utter disbelief. Why hadn't he told me about that before? Damaged muscle? It looked like a giant egg protruding from the pit of his arm. Bill just shrugged his shoulders.

After both doctors had examined him, feeling for lumps in his neck and stomach, the main doctor began discussing the films, pointing out irregularities in his bone marrow and necrosis in his shoulder bone. He ordered a biopsy of the armpit lump and another MRI. They both smiled and shook our hands as they left. My heart sank, but I tried to stay strong. Bill became talkative. And his feelings of guilt were obvious. He began telling me he simply didn't think the lump was anything worth mentioning to me.

Bill

Three months earlier, I had changed my weight-lifting routine. My trainer had me lifting heavier weights. During one of the first sessions, I pulled a muscle. Later I discovered the armpit lump and thought it was a result of the pulled muscle. Of course I didn't think it was cancer. Who would have? None of the symptoms discussed that day would have caused me to believe I had cancer. Of course I sweated a lot. I was an athlete living with a woman who was always cold and turning up the temperature in the house. Shoulder pain was a natural part of being a swimmer whose main stroke is the butterfly. Yes, I was tired, but who isn't these days? I worked full time and I was the father of two small children, a volunteer coach and very involved in many other activities. I was healthy and I was in great physical condition so how was it possible that I had cancer? People with cancer are supposed to be sick.

We left the orthopedic center and headed to Diagnostic Imaging to have an ultrasound. I was escorted back to a small room, asked to take off my shirt and lie down on a gurney. The nurse asked if I'd ever had an ultrasound before and I said "no". She said it wouldn't hurt. They were just going to take pictures of the lump. I put my arm over my head as the nurse rubbed the wand up and down my armpit. Then the doctor came in and did the same thing while also taking measurements and pictures of the lump. I got dressed and went back to the orthopedic center where we retrieved my schedule for the biopsy to be done the next morning.

On the way home, I was in a daze. It was all very overwhelming. I nervously anticipated the next day. I had never had a biopsy before and had no idea how they would do the procedure. Would they cut me open and remove the lump? All I wanted was for this whole thing to be over with so I could get back to training. I missed swimming and weights and being active and it had only just begun.

The next day, we returned to Diagnostic Imaging and signed in. This time, I asked if Dana-Susan could accompany me because I didn't want to be alone.

Dana-Susan

The procedure was down in the basement area. It was darker down there (at least it felt that way). We walked into a tiny room and Bill was instructed to get up on the gurney. A very funny nurse talked on and on about her family and how cold it was down there. It was nice seeing Bill laugh and flirt with her, behaving like himself. Another nurse came in and both ladies hooked him up to the monitor. Later, two doctors entered, one of whom was a fellow there to learn more about the procedure. A long needle was to be inserted into his lump. A sonogram camera monitored the procedure and guided the needle. The main doctor talked all the way through the process for the sake of the fellow, but Bill and I were quite fascinated by it all too. That was probably a good distraction from the fear of what we were facing. Throughout all of this, I thought us very fortunate to be getting such a great education.

As they began, I kept looking into Bill's eyes wondering if he felt pain. He smiled awkwardly and assured me he was pain-free, just a little uncomfortable. The monitor showed the inside of this lump which was now obviously not too small. Tissue was removed and they all prepared to make their many slides. Almost immediately the nurse came back to inform us we could rule out thyroid cancer. "Oh good," smiled Bill in great relief. I wondered why on Earth he was so happy to hear that when there were many other kinds of cancers and we'd never suspected that one anyway. I guess ruling out any cancer is good to hear when you're frightened.

So we'd done the blood work and the biopsy and it was time to head home and wait. That wait wasn't so bad. The results came back quickly. According to the pathologist, Bill had lymphoma, maybe follicular, but that's all we knew. More tests were ordered including bone scans, PET scan, bone marrow biopsies and CT scans. We spent much of our time at that cancer clinic. Our friends and family were calling, curious about his diagnosis. Many of them started searching "follicular lymphoma" on in the Internet. I wished they would stop. Reading little bits about a disease on the internet doesn't exactly make you an expert.

"I heard it's real simple to treat," some would say.

"Oh, lymphoma's not a bad cancer," one lady told me, "I have a friend who had Hodgkin's disease and he didn't even have to do chemo." I wondered if that lady would have felt so peaceful about it if her husband were facing lymphoma.

I know our friends only wanted to help, but I didn't want to hear their thoughts. I wanted to know what the lymphoma doctor had to say and we wouldn't see him for a couple of weeks.

My parents had been living in Spain, but had come to the States only two days before we heard that Bill had cancer. Without hesitation, they told me that they would be there for us during this time. My dad had commitments in Europe and would return for short visits, leaving my mom with me. She said from the beginning that her job was to take care of me and my children while I took care of my husband. While I considered myself Bill's source of strength and comfort, I realized quickly that my mom was mine. Her presence in our home was soothing.

Finally, it was time to hear the complete diagnosis. With great anticipation about the day, Bill and I sat in the exam room in the Lymphoma/Myeloma Clinic at MD Anderson. We chatted quietly, awaiting the doctor and the results of all the tests. Two weeks before, when this all began, I prayed for God to give my husband the perfect doctor. Being that we were at MD Anderson, I knew he would have an expert in lymphoma, but I wasn't going to settle for just another brilliant oncologist. I wanted perfect.

From the moment Dr. Fredrick Hagemeister walked into the room, I knew he was the right doctor for Bill. He shook our hands and looked into our eyes, looking at me as often as Bill. Before he even talked to us about the report, he said that now wasn't the time for the emotional part. Now we were there to hear the diagnosis and talk about treatments. He even looked at me and told me not to feel guilt about anything. I'm not really sure why he said that. Is that something he says to all his patients' spouses? But I liked it because later I would wonder if I'd given Bill some kind of virus to cause this disease. Remembering Dr. Hagemeister's words, I chose not to walk in guilt, but to deal with the way things were no matter the cause.

As we sat in that room hearing the details and extent of the disease, I don't know how we managed not to break down. Here was this lymphoma doctor telling us the very grim truth that my husband's body was riddled with cancer. The diagnosis: follicular lymphoma, stage four, grade three, extensively involving bone marrow. At least 90% of his bone marrow had been replaced by lymphoma. There was rare bone metastasis which had caused the bones in his shoulders, ribs and hips to die. And there were large tumors in his neck, chest, abdomen and pelvis. Dr. Hagemeister explained this disease on a level even I could comprehend. Follicular lymphoma, a type of non-Hodgkin lymphoma, is usually an indolent, slow-growing disease and it had become aggressive after possibly many years. He said Bill had likely had cancer for a decade without our knowing it. I sat there thinking how strange it was that on the day we got married and I vowed to love my husband in sickness and in health, he was standing before me with cancer.

"I think we'll do CHOP," said Dr. Hagemeister confidently. I could only assume that was some kind of chemo. Then he started talking about rituximab. I'd heard that word out in the waiting area as other patients were talking about it. I wasn't sure what it was, but from the sound of it, it was new and helped somehow with chemo. Soon, I would know more about this monoclonal antibody than I ever imagined. "Yes, CHOP," he said again, "We'll get this in remission."

Bill makes me laugh sometimes. Of course, he's an athlete and loves his fitness program. Here's a cancer doctor telling him he's got stage four of an aggressive blood cancer and his first question is "can I still run, swim and lift weights?" Well, here's how I knew this doctor was the perfect one for Bill. Although he told him he would not be able to do much other than walking due to the bone involvement, he smiled and said, "I'm a fitness fanatic too." I knew one thing for sure- this man was going to work hard to get my husband's cancer into remission. I liked everything about him from the beautiful tie he was wearing to the great resolve in his confident voice. There would eventually come a day when I realized he was one of my most favorite people I've ever met. We would learn that he truly and deeply cares about his patients. And he would someday become one of our most cherished friends.

When we left the clinic that day, we were exhausted. It had been a long, difficult morning that had dragged on into late afternoon. Bill was not able to start chemotherapy right away because one more test needed to be done. Also, he had chipped one of his teeth and the dental work needed to be done before chemo began. We phoned our family dentist on the way back to The Woodlands, a 45-minute drive north. His office was closing, but he would stay and wait for Bill and do whatever needed to be done as quickly as possible for him to start treatments. I dropped Bill off at the dentist. Everyone in the office was so kind, smiling at us. I could tell they felt sorry for us and for the first time, I realized that's how people would be looking at us from now on. It would be hard to get used to that.

I left Bill in the hands of the dentist and his team and went home to be with my mom and kids. My mom hugged me and suddenly I felt like a child again in her arms. I was 33 years old, but at that moment I felt like a five-year-old and like I could cry. I did not. Instead, I phoned a friend who was anxiously awaiting the results of Bill's tests. Then I called a family friend who is a physician and asked him to come over for dinner. I wanted him to look at the report and ask if he knew anything about CHOP.

When I picked Bill up from the dentist, I thought how I'd never seen him look so weary. He barely spoke. What was going on in his mind?

Bill

I continued to feel like this was all some kind of horrible mistake. It seemed like I was trapped in a bad dream and couldn't escape. Part of me wondered why I should be getting this tooth fixed if I was going to die. Why would I need a good tooth? But the bigger part of me wanted to hurry and get this done so I could start chemo and lick this cancer. The fighter was rising up in me. I wanted to get this disease in remission and quick. I wanted to get my life back and quick. Somehow, deep inside, I knew it wouldn't be that quick and easy.

The dentist told me how he'd had other chemo patients and gave me good suggestions for keeping my teeth clean during treatments. He and his staff tried to comfort me through the next hour, telling me they believed I'd be fine. I politely listened to them all, but found myself just escaping inside. Over the past couple of weeks, I'd been in shock. Now I was just as numb emotionally as my mouth was physically.

Dana-Susan

Our physician friend, Roger, arrived and we sat down for dinner. Then the phone rang. It was my brother-in-law's number. "I can't," Bill said. I understood and took the call myself in our room. Telling Bill's little brother the complete diagnosis was not too bad. I honestly wasn't sure whether he was more concerned about Bill or himself. Now he's had a sister die of leukemia and a brother diagnosed with lymphoma. I'd be wondering too. Moments later, my mother-in-law phoned. For many reasons, I found that call quite distressing and I had to dig deep inside to find the strength to handle it. We had been estranged and that was hard enough, but more difficult was realizing the enormity of telling a woman who has already lost a daughter to cancer that another of her children has cancer and that it's pretty bad.

She cried through the conversation, telling me she would try not to cry in front of Bill. For a moment I think she forgot he was an adult and was taken right back to the time her six-year-old little girl was dying and she was trying to be brave. "Tell Billy we'll be there for him through it all," she cried. After that call, I felt certain we would need extra grace to get through the greatest challenge of our lives!

We knew we would have to find a way of telling our kids. Morgan was five years old and Dylan was three. How would we put all of this on their level? We didn't have time to search for books and resources to explain cancer right away, so we would have to figure it all out on our own. Bill was so quiet. He wasn't sharing his feelings with anyone, including me. I knew he was trying hard to soak it all in and remain calm and positive and I knew he didn't want to scare the kids by breaking down, so it was up to me to explain this disease.

This was no time for lies. Bill and I asked the kids to sit on the couch. By the looks on their faces, I could tell they knew it wasn't good news we were there to share. "We have something to tell you that's not easy or good," I said. Bill held Dylan and Morgan sat by my side. They were quiet. "Daddy is sick. He has a disease called cancer," I said. "Cancer is not like having a cold. It's bigger than that. Daddy will have to go to the hospital a lot and take lots of medicine to try to make the cancer go away. The medicine is called chemotherapy and it does strange things to people." I slowly explained how chemo sometimes makes people's hair fall out. "Isn't that weird," I smiled trying to keep them from having fear. They were fascinated that their dad might be bald. I told them their dad would no longer be swimming with them because the doctor was going to put a catheter into his chest and it couldn't get wet. Bill told them he would not be able to coach swimming or soccer for a while so he could work on getting better. We did our best to be honest, while not scaring them. At the end of the talk, I asked if they understood what we said. Dylan answered, "I understand we need to pray for Daddy." Morgan looked down sadly and then into her daddy's eyes and said, "I understand perfectly." I was sure that was true.

That next night, Bill went to bed at 7:00 and shortly after, so did the kids. It was a lonely night and just the beginning of many lonely nights which lay ahead. I pulled out the photo albums and flipped through the pages of the early years of our marriage. There was my handsome husband coaching the swim team. I closed my eyes and thought about how I loved watching him do the butterfly stroke. His chest was always so strong and perfectly sculpted. When I saw him fly in the pool, I melted. His strength and grace were amazing. "Will I ever get to see my Bill do the butterfly stroke again", I thought. Then I sat on the floor, photo albums clutched to my chest, and had my first cry.

After that night, I would cry some again, but not much. Others around me cried for me. Somehow their tears strengthened me and I was thankful for the ones willing to show their sorrow. One morning at church, some people prayed for us. A lady beside me cried bitterly. As each of her tears fell forcefully on her Bible, it seemed like more strength was added to me. It was as if she was taking my burden from me. She and many others wept for Bill and our family, flooding Heaven with prayer.

A time to kill...

Dana-Susan

*D*ays later, all the tests complete, we returned to the clinic and headed to Infusion Therapy. A central venous catheter was to be inserted in Bill's chest with a line to the main vein in his heart. Through this PICC line, chemo would be infused and blood would be drawn. We had attended a pre-op class to learn how the procedure is done and learned it was quite simple. It would take about 20 minutes to insert and then an X-ray would be done to ensure it was inserted into the right vein.

That day, Bill was to have the CVC line inserted and following, we would attend another class in which I would learn how to care for it at home. The waiting room was packed that morning, but I finally found a place to sit. Bill was escorted by a nurse to his room while I waited. A television was on and soon they were reporting on national news the horrible Houston weather. Reports of tornadoes and flooding all over the city got me a little nervous. How were we going to get home? An hour passed and still I heard nothing from Bill. I wondered what was taking so long and began to get even more frustrated about the horrible weather. Another hour passed and I really began to wonder. "They said it would take 20 minutes and he's been gone two hours", I thought. Then a nurse came out and called, "Mrs. Crews, wife of William Crews." There was no doubt something wasn't right. "Your husband needs you," she said.

As the nurse escorted me to the exam room, I felt shaky. But I was determined to be that rock for Bill, so I took a deep breath and prayed for strength. Nothing could have prepared me for the ugly picture I saw when that door was opened. My husband was lying on a gurney, his carved up chest exposed. Blood was covering the white sheets and pain was in his eyes. I walked slowly to him and kissed his forehead. "It hurts bad," he quietly spoke. His voice was scratchy. A few minutes later, the head surgeon, a charming man, entered the room. He explained to me what had gone wrong. They simply were not accustomed to patients having such a muscular chest. "All those years of the beautiful butterfly stroke", I thought. One of the doctors had attempted to force the line into his chest but it would not go through all his muscle and began to get caught in his throat. Now that explained why his voice was so scratchy. Finally the head surgeon told her to give it up. They were awaiting a call from Bill's doctor to give permission to put the line into his arm instead.

That call finally came and permission was granted. Then another person came in to prep him to have the CVC line put in his arm. This time it was what they called a "long line" because it had to be long enough to go from just above his right wrist, up through his arm and shoulder and down into the vein in his heart. As she prepped him, I sat on a stool while the head surgeon obviously tried to distract me with stories about his daughter who was traveling in Africa. I half-way listened and kept my eyes on Bill who was obviously in great pain. Before my eyes, his chest turned black. I thought that if I could imagine the pain, it would be like I was taking it from him. "Feel the pain", I thought, "feel the pain". I cringed as they poked through his arm and the long line once again refused to go into the right place. "I keep hitting blood vessels," said the nurse. Bill's face revealed it all. He hurt. But he was tough and endured it to the end.

Bill

When I was told that I would have to have a CVC line put in my chest, I really did not understand what it meant. We went to that first orientation class, and I realized how much my life was being taken away from me. The dummy they used to show us where the CVC line was going to be placed had two IV lines hanging out of its chest. These lines hung down about two inches. My first thought was "how will I take a shower with that in my chest?" I had no idea what would be involved in taking care of these lines as we had not been to the care classes yet. At this point however, I was ready to begin the fight. I felt the sooner we got started, the sooner this would be over.

I was a little anxious in the infusion therapy waiting room, waiting to be called back for this simple catheter insertion. When they called me back, I was escorted to a small procedure room where a doctor and nurse had me lie down on a gurney. They told me that this should only take about twenty minutes and then I would be out for an X-ray. They explained the technicalities of how they were going to start by deadening a small spot on my chest and then as they proceeded to thread the catheter into my veins, if there was any discomfort, they could give me more local anesthetic. The doctor said that she expected the head of surgery to stop by in a little while as he was supposed to observe her that day. Then we started.

The initial deadening of the skin went fine. Then it seemed everything went downhill. First she could not find the correct vein to put the catheter in. So she had to pull it out and start over. Then, she found a vein, but could not get the catheter to turn the correct way. It ended up snaking over my throat. The process of trying to insert this catheter into my chest continued for two hours. The local anesthetic wore off several times during this. Finally, the head of surgery walked in, saw all the blood, and put a stop to the mutilation of my chest. He immediately told me and the attending doctor that he was going to call my doctor and ask if the catheter could be put in my arm instead. If my doctor did not agree to this, he explained that I would have to go through a more complicated surgery using the ultrasound machine for guidance of the CVC line.

As he left the room, I asked if Dana-Susan could come in. She was the person I wanted to see more than anyone else in the world. I was in great pain and knew that she could bring me comfort. I had been separated from her for over two hours now, even though this was only supposed to be a 20-minute procedure. As she walked in the room and over to me, I knew that everything would be fine again. I hate that she had to see me so vulnerable, but I needed her. Soon the head surgeon came back and said they were going to put the line into my arm. The nurse then bandaged my chest and started prepping my arm. Again, this was supposed to be a quick procedure. They allowed Dana-Susan to stay in the room this time. The head of surgery also stayed in the room and kept up small talk with Dana-Susan as they worked on me. Soon it was obvious this was not going well as they had to start over several times. An hour later, they were taking me to X-ray finally as the catheter was inserted and they had to be sure it had gone in the right artery. Dana-Susan attended her catheter care class as I went to X-ray alone.

Dana-Susan

So, a simple 20-minute procedure had turned into three hours of excruciating pain and vast complications. As they rolled Bill away into X-ray, I attended the CVC care class. I sat in a wooden school desk surrounded by other caregivers and patients. A kind nurse walked in, handed us all a booklet, a pencil for notetaking, and a catheter and care kit. Most of the patients in the room had just had their catheters inserted and I saw fear in their eyes. The caregivers had a different kind of fear in their eyes, and I wondered if I looked just like all of them. We were all facing the same uncertainties. We were all being forced into a world of disease, destruction and possible death. Soon, a video began, and we all watched a woman clean and dress her husband's suture site. Then the nurse got out a dummy and began to demonstrate it again. I learned how to flush his catheter with an anticoagulant (blood thinner) every 24 hours and how to change the dressing twice each week. I learned how to check for infections which could be life-threatening. Bill finally joined me, looking exhausted. He sat next to me as I began to practice flushing and dressing on the catheter on my desk.

When I saw Bill this time, he looked worse than I'd ever seen him. I was so used to having a happy, healthy husband. Seeing him so weak and tired and in such agony was troublesome. He began to feel nauseated and headachy. In one more hour his appointment with Dr. Hagemeister was on the schedule.

The waiting area in the Lymphoma/Myeloma clinic was packed. It was standing room only. Apparently the amount of patients with blood cancers was growing as rapidly as the cancer in my husband's body. The receptionist brought out extra chairs for us. I asked them if Bill could leave for a while to rest in the comfy recliners in the patient area downstairs. But they thought it a bad idea because we might miss the appointment. They explained that the doctor was leaving the next morning for a conference in Tokyo where he would be speaking about new treatments for lymphoma.

Just as I had expected, the short one-hour wait became close to three hours. All that time, Bill's chest and arm were pounding as was his head and he began to get a migraine. I continued to be distressed by the cruel weather. I looked out the windows and saw black skies and hail, rising waters and thought how that nasty weather matched the dark, cold emotion inside me. "Should we think about staying here at the hotel," I asked Bill. "No," came a quick, sharp answer. I knew he was in great agony.

Bill

My head was pounding. My shoulder was in agony and I was feeling angry at the doctor who'd just spent three hours butchering my chest. All I wanted was to get home. I wanted to crawl up in my own bed and sleep. I thought Dana-Susan was over-reacting about the weather even though the news was reporting tornadoes and hailstorms with flooding. I didn't really care at that moment about anything but escaping my pain. Soon a full-blown migraine hit and I knew it would only get worse.

Dana-Susan

Dr. Hagemeister quickly went over the latest test results which didn't change the diagnosis or treatments he'd intended. Bill was going to be doing R-CHOP, eight cycles. Later we would talk about future treatments after re-staging. We said goodbye to the good doctor and waited for his nurse to bring us educational materials about chemotherapy. She had us watch a quick video about chemo in which we learned about side effects. Moments before, Dr. Hagemeister had already explained those side effects and I was trying hard not to let fear enter my mind. He had told us there were three groups of side effects: first were the things that were not likely to happen, but likely to kill you such as heart failure, liver or kidney failure. Then there were the things that were likely to happen, but not likely to kill you such as hair loss, nausea and fatigue. Then there were the things that were likely to happen and likely to kill you (and here's where I had to control my fear instead of letting it control me) – infections.

By the time our video was over and we'd read through the educational materials, it was 5:00 in the evening. Although we had fully expected Bill to begin treatments that day, it was obviously not happening. Rituximab would be the first drug infused and it would take up to eight hours to infuse. Besides it being so late, the pharmacist had a disagreement with the prescription and we would have to wait and have that sorted out. Nurse Judy told us to go home and wait to hear from them first thing in the morning.

As we walked toward the sky bridge, I once again pleaded with Bill to let us stay in the hotel right across the street. It was so very dark outside, and the streets were flooded. "No," he demanded, "get me home." His head and chest were throbbing.

We walked out into the harsh weather. It was still pouring rain and for 5:00 was quite dark. Traffic lights had been blown out and traffic was backed up for miles. Driving is not something I like even in good conditions. I wondered how I would get home with the many streets shut down. Bill crawled into the back of our SUV and begged me to get him home quickly. It wasn't possible. The freeway was flooded, and the streets were packed with traffic and noise. I couldn't see. I didn't know any alternate routes home and had to just find any street without flood waters. Eventually I made my way to the only open road and looked to the access roads where I saw people on top of their vehicles waiting to be rescued by boat. I turned on the radio and listened to the news. All over the city, power was out and people were being rescued. Mighty winds shook our large SUV.

Rising waters scared me and I couldn't imagine driving through them. We had left home that morning at 5:30 and here we were 12 hours later in a black storm, the end nowhere in sight. Bill had been tortured that day and his body was eaten up with cancer. He was in the back in excruciating pain and I was in rising flood waters with wind and hailstorms and tornadoes surrounding me. Suddenly Bill sat up in the back, put the window down and began to vomit. Bye brave, strong Dana-Sue! I had my second big cry and one of the loneliest, most stressful night I'd ever known. My protective husband who would have never wanted me to be driving in this kind of storm, was now uncontrollably vomiting out the window and completely unaware of what was happening. I phoned my mom crying into the phone. She talked to me and tried to comfort me, but I could tell she was feeling pretty concerned about us. I turned on soft music thinking it would calm me. It didn't, but soon Bill was asleep in the back. That was good for him, but I felt so alone.

Four hours later, we were home, rains still pouring from the black skies. Once again, the storms of life encompassed us that day and night. This time, though, it felt like we were each facing them on our own. I helped Bill out of the car and into the house where my mom and daughter grabbed me and held me. "I'm tired," I softly said.

We slept for a few hours that night and woke up still not knowing when the appointment for treatments would begin. They said they would call first thing in the morning, but that was not true. What we knew for sure that morning was that we had to return to Infusion Therapy to have Bill's catheter checked and for me to demonstrate for the nurse I could take care of it myself at home. His chest and arm were black, and he was slightly "hungover" from the migraine the night before. We waited and waited, but no one from the lymphoma clinic called. Bill tried calling them with no luck. He tried again and again. I also tried calling, but we were told only to wait. They would call when they had the schedule ready. All we knew was that the doctor was leaving that morning for Tokyo and that the pharmacist had not approved the chemo prescription. "What happens if the doctor leaves and it doesn't get sorted out", I thought. "Will Bill die waiting for chemo?"

Late that morning, we returned to Infusion Therapy and on the way, Nurse Judy phoned to tell us treatments were definitely being scheduled, but she didn't know what time yet. At Infusion Therapy, we waited for a while before a very gracious nurse brought us to her room where she would "test" me. I slowly removed the bandages from Bill's arm and was stunned to see the damage. It was so terribly bruised. No wonder he had all that pain. And his chest was even worse. Very carefully I cleaned his suture site and changed the dressing. I passed my test and we left once again for the lymphoma clinic to see when they'd scheduled the chemo. Bill asked to see Nurse Judy, giving the receptionist his name. Ten minutes later, she came out and said, "I couldn't remember who you were and then I said, 'oh, yes, the young man with a whole lot of cancer'."

That wasn't pretty. But it was true. After a long wait, Nurse Judy got the paperwork in order and we were off to have lunch before heading to the Ambulatory Treatment Center for Round One of R-CHOP. While we sat in the waiting area, I glanced at Bill who seemed far away. I could only imagine his fear. Was he thinking about his sister and her battle against cancer? Or maybe, and more likely, was he thinking of his good friend Chad? Chad had been a great friend to Bill and had suffered leukemia in these very halls for two long years. Bill had said how he wished he could talk to Chad.

Bill

I wished I could talk to someone who'd been in my shoes. I wondered what it would be like to have chemo working its way through my body. How would my body react? Would I get sick? If only I could talk to someone, anyone who'd done this before. I was extremely nervous going into the great unknown.

My friend Chad came to mind. Only a few months before, he'd fought for his life right here in this place. Perhaps he'd even sat in this exact chair with his wife Cindy by his side. I remembered the last time I'd seen Chad. He was bald and so frail and I wondered if the chemo would have that same effect on me. Chad was only 31, but he looked like an old man. Cancer and chemo had eaten his life away. Was that my fate too?

Dana-Susan

"William Crews, Jr.," called the nurse. It was 3:00 by that time. We were taken to the room where they weighed him and took his blood pressure. Then he was assigned his room number. It was a nice, private room with a bed and chair and television. We got settled and soon they were bringing Bill Tylenol and Benadryl. I wasn't quite sure I understood it all, but I knew that rituximab, a monoclonal antibody made of mouse and human proteins, could cause allergic reactions. We didn't have a lot of time in the two weeks since we'd discovered Bill had cancer to truly study the disease or treatments like we wanted. Quickly we looked over the few resources we had about the drugs and knew that rituximab was still fairly new. It had only recently still been in clinical trial phase.

Rituximab is a therapy that looks for B cells, where Bill's cancer originated. B cells are found in the blood and lymph nodes and have a protein on their cell wall called CD20. Rituximab looks for that protein, attaches to cells that have it and destroys them. It uses the body's own immune system to help it kill B cells. Using it with standard chemotherapy was supposedly going to help patients achieve long term remission.

Before the infusion began, the nurse administered bags of saline and made sure we understood the potential side effects. Although we acknowledged we did, the truth was we could only imagine, and our imagination was nothing compared to reality. When she pushed the button and Bill's first chemo infusion had begun, it was quite surreal. Within 15 minutes, his body was violently shaking and covered in hives. He shook so much, he was falling off the bed so I grabbed him after calling for the nurse. He was so cold. The nurse rushed in and stopped the infusion. He had definitely reacted to the drug. We would have to stop for a while, then start again at a much slower rate. She then gave him more Benadryl and a bag of Demerol was pumped into his body. When he continued to react, more Demerol was infused. He was loaded down with drugs, and I was loaded down with sorrow. I hated this. It was not fun and I wanted someone to tell me it was all some kind of bad dream and I would soon wake up and we'd be swimming laps together and riding bikes through the trails.

Hours and hours passed slowly by in the chemo unit that night. Bill was weak and weary and barely able to speak. I was cold and tired. My mind had been filled with thoughts of cancer and chemo for days and I needed a small break. I was introduced to reality television that night. The show I watched was about Paris Hilton and Nicole Richey who were milking cows on a farm in Arkansas. It amused me while Bill was sleeping.

When finally the infusion was over, more than nine hours after it had begun, it was 1:00 a.m. This day had been much longer than I had expected. My neighbor who is a nurse had told me that often chemo patients get this thing called "chemo brain" and they don't think clearly. She told me that Bill and I needed a nice, easy word or phrase that would indicate to him that he wasn't thinking clearly and that I was doing the thinking at certain times. We chose "banana nut bread" and it signified that he needed to let me make the decision at the moment. He had been through hours of infusion of all kinds of drugs, including

Demerol and Benadryl and an allergic reaction to the antibody. It was 1:00 a.m. and he grabbed the keys and said "I'll drive home." I took the keys from him and sweetly said, "banana nut bread".

The next morning, we returned to the treatment center for the next three drugs to be infused. I could not have imagined ever being this tired. Would it be like this for the next several months? Would we ever get any rest? The first of the chemotherapy drugs began to infuse. It took an hour and a half. Bill looked fine and didn't react at all. Immediately, the next drug was administered. He still had no reactions. It took about half an hour. Then the nurse came in with the third bag of chemo and a portable pump. This last drug was so potent and there was so much of it that it required a 48-hour infusion so we were instructed on how to disconnect it at home. Bill would wrap this chemo in a bag around his waist sort of like a fanny pack and after it dripped for two days, I would disconnect it and clean him up. We would return to the clinic to turn in the pump later. As the nurse demonstrated the pump and its alarm, she brought out the bag of chemo. All the other drugs, including the rituximab the night before had been clear in color. If we had wanted to, we could have pretended they weren't chemo at all, but maybe a simple saline or something. This last one was red. A big, bright red bag of poison! Later we would learn that its nickname amongst other patients was "Red Devil" and we knew why almost instantly.

The nurse hooked him up and started the drip. In less than a minute, Bill already felt the burning sensation mixed with nausea. While it began, the nurse explained the potency of this drug. "When you disconnect," she said, "you have to wear your gloves and change the cap and dressing over a disposable towel. If even a tiny drop of this drug gets on your skin, it could severely burn your flesh."

I was trying to imagine how a chemical toxic enough to severely burn my flesh was so steadily going into the main vein to my husband's heart.

Bill

Immediately after the pump started, I could feel a burning in my chest. It felt like boiling liquid was dropping down into my heart. Then, for some reason, I got hiccups. That would happen every time that drug was infused and wouldn't stop for 48 hours. I also began to feel nausea within the first couple of minutes. I told the nurse and she reminded me to begin taking my anti-nausea medicine.

Finally, I felt frightened. The first drugs were nothing compared to this one. I began to wonder about all the possibilities. I wondered how I would sleep with this chemo wrapped around my waist. I wondered what would happen if the tubing broke and chemo spilled out all over the bed. I decided right then I would be sleeping on the couch so it wouldn't harm my wife. I wondered if I'd be losing my hair soon.

Thanksgiving was coming up. I'd been told that days nine

through 15 of this chemo cycle would be when my counts would be at their lowest. I wondered if I would be able to enjoy the holiday with family or if I'd have to be isolated. My mind was filled with unanswerable questions. This was a battle I would have to fight out one step at a time, and it was just as much mental and emotional as it was physical.

That night, I slept a little. I felt so sick. When I woke up, Dana-Susan was there asking how I felt. I mumbled a quick answer and turned to see her wiping my hair off the pillow. It had already started falling out. Dana-Susan got the clippers and asked, "Do you want the chemo to take your hair or do you want the kids to do it?" Nervously, I chose the kids.

Before that treatment, I had fantasized that maybe I would be able to escape the effects of chemotherapy. Maybe I would just breeze through it. That fantasy was over. I was already weak and sick and the first treatment wasn't even over. Cancer was bad. Chemo was worse. How would I manage to endure this horrible mess for eight cycles?

A time of war...

Bill

*D*uring the many months of intensive chemotherapy, I went through many highs and lows mentally, emotionally and physically. There were times when I'd sleep for days as I was exhausted from chemo and fighting cancer. Other times, I felt like I had so much energy I was going to burst if I couldn't go out and do something. And I couldn't do the kinds of activities I'd always done. My body was fighting even when my mind and spirit couldn't fight. Someone told me that the best thing I could do for my body was to take it on daily walks just to fight the fatigue. Of all the side effects, that one was the worst. I hated being weary. But I gave walking a try and did it when I could. It made me feel like I had some power and control over this disease and I wasn't going to let it completely destroy my life.

As I walked alone, I would think and pray. I'd never go too far from the house because I feared I might not have the energy to return home. It was while out on one of these walks one afternoon, that something changed in me. I felt God's presence that day. It was as if He was reassuring me that He had purpose in allowing this disease into my life and that He would safely bring me through. With God on my side, my fears began to fade.

Although I was mostly weary during these months, deep inside me there was a soldier battling sickness and death. I even had a vivid dream one night that Jesus was by my side, grabbing a sword, handing me one, and the two of us stood together fighting cancer cells. It encouraged me to keep fighting and to stay alive. I wanted to live. I was a dad and a husband. My wife and my children are my great love, and I couldn't bear the thought of leaving them alone.

I would not give in to death. If I died, I would go down fighting. That's what Chad did. That's what my sister did. That's what many others do. In the end, some people live, and some people die. What makes us all the same is we fight hard to live and hope the treatments work. I was fortunate to have a family fighting by my side. My wife and kids fought the cancer all in their own ways. Without fail, Dana-Susan remembered to flush my cap every 24 hours. Even if I fell asleep, she'd sneak in and flush it. Twice a week, she cleaned and dressed my catheter. After the dressing, she initialed the bandage and drew a little heart beside it. She kept everything clean and sterile. My towels were all bleached and my clothes were cleaned in the hottest water. I knew she was working extra hard to keep out the germs. She was a great nurse.

Morgan and Dylan were little champions in this war on cancer. It was tough on them, but they endured. I was honored to have them fight on my side. I didn't always show my gratitude, but I was touched to my core by the act of love from my beautiful family. I include my mother-in-law in this. She was a mom to us all and none of us could have survived without her.

Dana-Susan

We were determined to maintain an overall spirit of joy and

laughter in our home, no matter what. If our first weapon against this disease was prayer, our second weapon was joy. We found reasons to be happy and to laugh. In the chemo unit, Bill and I laughed at magazine articles or funny movies. For the hours and hours we waited in hospital waiting rooms, we wrote "top 10 lists" and told jokes. Yes, we were a little twisted and discovered "tumor humor". But we weren't alone in that. Other patients did the same and we quickly bonded with the cancer community.

It was weird because I will never forget the first time we were waiting for Bill to have a bone scan. We sat in the lobby and when they finally called his name along with two other men, the three of them got up and headed down the long hall. I sat there with the other wives watching as our husbands slowly made their way down the long, empty hall. It struck me that morning as I noticed how good-looking and fit Bill was and I thought, "You've got the wrong guy!"

But somehow, over time, I stopped thinking that. Cancer became a natural and normal part of our lives. Oh, I didn't just sit there and take it, accepting it and welcoming it with open arms. I hated and continue to hate cancer. But I learned to fight it by embracing the good work it was doing in us. We became a part of that "cancer club" and even learned to be thankful for it. When they called Bill, I no longer felt misplaced like I was living someone else's life. I felt like I belonged right there by his side in this community. MD Anderson had once seemed like the most awful place on Earth. But it had now become a second home and I fell in love with it. Where once I had seen darkness and death, I now saw hope and life. Bill said he loved it there because they didn't have a "defeatist attitude". Right! I could feel that. The brave men, women and children who walked those halls were champions. They fought with courage against their diseases and refused to give in. So the atmosphere was uplifting and proved that even when facing death, you don't have to cower to it. And not only were the patients filled with great valor, but their caregivers were as well. I saw sweet old ladies carefully wheel their dying husbands through the long halls and endlessly love on them. I saw young married couples in their twenties holding hands in the waiting rooms, young husbands wrapping their cancer-stricken young wives up in warm blankets and fetching them hot tea. Although I didn't usually make it to the pediatric unit, I often saw precious children holding their parents' hands as they made their way through the halls. Their smiling faces revealed incredible courage. I began to write in my journal about the many brave warriors I met or saw in this amazing institution.

When I saw a small girl in the gift shop one day, I was inspired by her smile. She sat quietly in a wheel chair with a pink blanket draped over her legs. Her bald head was exposed and a huge scar ran from one side to the other. Her mom was showing her a card and they both laughed. I thought about the young mother and how harsh this was for her. But I mostly thought about the light in that young child's eyes. Her little face glowed. She was one of many, many people, young and old, who lit up the halls of that hospital and made the battle ground of this war so rich with hope.

None of that made this war against cancer any easier. And I do call it a war because when cancer happens, it feels like a terrorist has attacked. I hated the pain and sickness. I hated it when Bill had bone marrow aspirations and limped around for days following. Having them drill a hole into his hip bone to suck out the marrow was unbearable. Watching my best friend get sicker each day, seeing his skin grow paler and his once solid muscles turn to thin frailty – none of that was fun. And when he lost his hair, it wasn't like it looks in the movies. He wasn't just bald. He lost his eyebrows and lashes and every part of his body that once had hair, no longer did. His face went through periods of thinness and then puffiness depending on which stage of the chemo cycle he was in. It was all very intense and truly overwhelming. But part of the process was winning the war on my attitude.

When his hair started falling out, we didn't want the drugs to win, so we got out the clippers and let Morgan and Dylan shave his head. Bill was pretty nervous, afraid they might chop off his ear. But I closely monitored, and we made going bald a fun family affair. Somehow, we made cancer a family affair and used it to draw us closer and make us better. Those are just some of the many ways we won the war. That's why I knew that even if cancer took my husband's life, it wouldn't win the war because even in his death, we would be victorious, continuing to wage war against it for others in his honor.

I could never say I love cancer because I don't, but I am thankful it came into our lives. I am thankful that I got the privilege to see my husband stand up to it and fight with strength, confidence and faith to beat it. I'm thankful I saw my children filled with courage, fighting their fears and growing in character even at an early age. I'm thankful for the people we met and for the opportunity to watch first-hand as men and women and children stood in the face of the monster cancer and defied it. It was and continues to be a great thrill.

Of course, there were days when I wanted to escape it. Brief moments would come and remind me of the life we once knew, and I would long for it. I would be sitting in the chemo unit watching Bill sleep and if I closed my eyes, I could almost smell chlorine and hear my children's laughter. I could see their joyful eyes as their daddy drove home from work in his Jeep and jumped out to greet them, full of energy and life. Then I'd open my eyes and it all quickly faded as instead of swimming pools and soccer fields I saw I.V. pumps and blood pressure machines and alcohol swabs.

Most of the time, I was fine. I had made a conscious decision in the very beginning not to think about the past or the future, but to live in the moment. If I thought too much about the past, I might grow bitter and resentful for everything I felt had been stolen from us. And the future, why, it was too uncertain. Better was to concentrate on the task at hand and deal with whatever moment I was in. If it was time to change the dressing on Bill's CVC line, I would concentrate on that job. If he was having chemo and needed me to fetch him water, I got up and did that.

I drove through traffic in the early morning, late at night and throughout the day, taking him to and from the medical center. If he was awake in the middle of the night vomiting, I would sit outside of the bathroom praying for him, comforting him when he came out. When he got borderline fevers, I monitored them closely. I bleached everything in sight trying to keep out all the impurities. My mind was focused on the immediate. Often, I didn't even realize how I felt about any of this. I was disconnected from my emotions and almost just running on autopilot.

By the time his treatments were over 2 ½ years later, that would present itself with its own problems as I would finally recognize the depth of emotional pain this disease had inflicted upon me. Meanwhile, I did what was necessary to help my husband and my children endure the many struggles in our family's fight against cancer.

One morning I awoke after a long, difficult night to hear Bill groaning. For some reason, he was having nausea, severe cramping and rectal bleeding. We weren't sure what to do, so we called the hospital. After being instructed to head to the emergency room at MD Anderson, I found childcare for the kids, and we began the 45-minute drive to Houston. Our wait wasn't long in the emergency room. A pretty, young doctor examined him and told Bill she thought it was nothing too serious but that he might need to have a colonoscopy eventually if it didn't cease. "So you get lymphoma and that puts you at risk for all other cancers", I wondered. It would turn out to be no big deal and the colonoscopy was never ordered. But that long morning and afternoon of once again spending hours and hours at the cancer clinic was in and of itself a huge stress. Although I didn't always recognize it, just being there going through this was causing distress and pain in me that would build up over time. I made the worst mistake I think a caregiver can make. Instead of seeking support from others who'd been in my shoes, I ignored my feelings and tried to "push through" just as I'd always done with my pain as an athlete. There were many support groups to join at the medical center, but I didn't want to be away from home if I didn't have to, so I toughed it out on my own. It ended up causing some harm to my health too. I no longer had time or energy to keep up my full fitness program. My diet turned to eating whatever I could whenever I could, or sometimes not eating at all. When we had time, I dragged Bill to Pilates or attended kickboxing, but it wasn't a daily program as it had always been. It didn't take long for my muscles to go. My body was thin and pale and I often thought were it not for the head full of hair, I'd look like a cancer patient myself.

Chemo brain was stealing Bill from me. Mostly he slept when he was home. I don't know how he continued to work, but he never quit his job or took extended time off. But by the time he was home, his energy was spent and he slept or laid on the couch in a daze. Many days and most nights, I felt like he was gone. I missed him. I'd catch myself thinking, "I wish Bill were here helping me take care of this cancer patient". Harder than that was the weird effect the drugs were having on his mind and emotions. Bill had always been very easy-going, not given to strange worry. But suddenly he was panicking about everything. Out of the blue he'd say things like, "I don't want you to cook anymore because I'm scared you'll catch on fire." Or "What will we do if our dishwasher breaks?" I wondered how he could be so concerned about a kitchen appliance he never used. His fears and confusion were tough to bear. But the worst trouble of all was the feeling that he was gone from my life and might never return.

We didn't talk much about the "what ifs". Because we were fighting so hard against this disease, we tried to keep a positive attitude that we'd beat it. Death was the ultimate enemy and we hoped to conquer it, but its possibility was hovering over us like a dark cloud. Even the kids could feel it. I will never forget that sinking feeling one evening while at our neighbor's home. We all sat around the table talking when suddenly Morgan got up, sat on her daddy's lap and kissed him all over his cheek before whispering in his ear, "Daddy, I'm giving you all my love because you might die." Bill was stunned and could barely speak.

Later in the night I held Morgan on her bed. We had never told the kids cancer killed people. Where did she get that idea? "Mommy, I know Daddy's sister died of cancer," she said, "so I figured it out. Daddy's got cancer and he might die." Now my heart sank. I sat looking into Morgan's sweet blue eyes as a tear rolled down her pretty round cheek. "Don't worry, Mom," she said, "If he dies, I know he'll go to Heaven."

Sometimes we're given opportunities for life lessons at an early age. Death and taxes are inevitable and now was the time for my precious little girl to know the truth. Death is part of life. We'd save the ugly truth about taxes for another day.

"You're right," I answered Morgan, "if Daddy dies, he will go to Heaven. But just because someone has cancer, that doesn't mean they are going to die." As I sat by my little girl's side, I told her how everyone dies. The difficulty is that any of us could die at any time and we don't know when our appointed time is. What's so amazing about life is that we can enjoy it here and now no matter what. There's no point in fretting over death. Instead, we should choose to enjoy life. All that was easy to say, but not quite as easy to live out. When I left Morgan, I knew she would be alright eventually, but I also knew she was battling out many emotions, struggling on her own just as I had been.

Dylan was so little, but the tension was getting to him too. Although we had tried with everything in us to maintain a positive attitude, the truth was we were up against a monster enemy, and it wore us all down. My three-year-old little guy was filled with courage beyond his years, but he suffered many nights from terrible dreams. He didn't quite comprehend the idea of death, but I could tell from the nightmares, this was profoundly affecting him too. He dreamed of being eaten up by lions or beaten by "bad guys". His torment was very real and as a mom, I felt extra burdened to fix everyone's troubles. The simple truth was, I couldn't. I had to be patient and find strength to get through each day. My children had to learn to do that too.

Facing adversity can produce good things if you let it. It can build mental, spiritual and emotional muscles and I got the beautiful opportunity to witness that first-hand in my husband, in my children and in me. Nothing was easy, but it was all used for good. Life continued the way life does. Troubles came and troubles went. We faced huge giants and beat them down. Yes we were all weary and wounded, but toughened up as a result. War is hell, they say, and I agree. But I'm thankful for the honor of being a soldier.

A time to heal...

Dana-Susan

*A*fter three months of intensive chemotherapy, Bill was re-staged. He had to do all the scans and biopsies again, none of them pleasant. Again, he endured hours of scans, including having to drink disgusting cocktails like berry-flavored Barium. More bone marrow aspirations. More blood work. Then the day came for us to hear how that chemo had worked. It was January 26, 2004 when we sat in the exam room awaiting the doctor, but instead a young fellow entered. He didn't speak English well and neither Bill nor I understood what he was saying. He went over the report without handing it to us and as he finished speaking, I thought, "Either Bill's got stage four lymphoma or he's in remission, but I can't tell".

Dr. Hagemeister then walked into the room and smiled, "You're in complete remission." I was shocked. I looked at Bill. He just sat there. "Why aren't you excited", I wondered. The doctor went over the report and he seemed very excited. And why not? He successfully got this 37-year-old lymphoma patient into complete remission and in only a few short months.

Bill

My first question when I heard I was in remission was "Do I still have to do chemo?" Sadly, the answer was yes. Then I asked if I could cut it short and only do six cycles. Again the answer was not what I wanted. No, I would have to finish all eight cycles and then do maybe two years of "maintenance" chemo. I guess that's the way it is with an incurable disease. At the time, I was only half-way finished with R-CHOP and in only an hour, I'd be back in the chemo unit having more poison pumped into me. Maybe that's why I wasn't jumping for joy. I was happy to be in remission and hopeful that I'd stay that way, but somehow I knew this battle wasn't over.

Dana-Susan

When we walked out to the hall to wait for the nurse to bring chemo orders, I phoned my mom. She and my dad were thrilled. Next, I phoned my boss and asked that she call all my coworkers. I had been teaching part-time at my kids' school, a private pre-school and kindergarten. I was the lead teacher for a toddler class as well as the Spanish teacher for the whole school. Although I was rarely at work, I went as often as possible because I thought it was good for my own two kids and I loved my precious students. Plus, some of the greatest ladies on Earth taught there. They, along with my mother, got me through this awful time. Their constant notes of encouragement, making us meals, caring for my children, sending flowers and special gifts were like a taste of Heaven. So the first ones to hear that Bill was in remission should be my mom and my teacher friends. They were all in celebration mode.

I was happy too, but feeling a little confused. For some reason, I couldn't dance a jig yet. An hour later, I realized why. Once again, we were in the chemo unit and I sat by my husband's side while poison pumped through his veins. The thought occurred to me that now that the chemo wasn't going to be killing cancer cells, it would be killing something. Would it kill Bill?

While in the chemo unit, I called one of Bill's friends. He, too, was excited to hear the news, but I liked his analogy. Perhaps it was because the Super Bowl was in a few days, but his made the most sense to me. "You're first and goal," he said. Bill and I were players on the field and it was now first and goal. Our fans (friends and family) were excited because all we had to do is get this goal and win the game, so they were clapping and shouting and dancing. Meanwhile, Bill and I had to finish the game and even though the possibility of winning seemed very likely, it wasn't a sure thing.

Getting through these next few months was not going to be easy. Bill grew weaker and weaker. Some days he seemed to barely cling to life. Nights were the toughest for me. Often I couldn't tell if he was breathing and would stay awake all night just to make sure he was alive. He experienced the many side effects his doctor warned him about, including nausea, some vomiting and fatigue, which was to him, the worst one of all. We also noticed burn marks on his skin from where the chemo had burned him from the inside out. Aside from four toxins being pumped into his body every three weeks, he was also taking a large dose of steroids, sleeping pills, anti-nausea medicine, Procrit shots and Neulasta. His body was full of drugs.

It was a dull, gray winter that year. It rained more than usual. Life was getting harder to live as troubles seemed to encompass us. We felt like we'd been through fires and floods and couldn't escape. Was the end in sight? And was the end good or bad? Through the winter months we held on to hope, but grew more and more weary. Spring was slow in arriving and unfortunately, did not bring with it health. Morgan had been suffering from ear infections for some time and finally it was inevitable. She would need surgery to have tubes in her ears and her adenoids removed. Sometimes I felt like our family was falling apart. Once we'd been known for our energy and athleticism. Now we were the sick people. It was March. Bill had two chemo treatments that month and sandwiched between them was Morgan's surgery. "I want a break", I thought. But that would not be happening.

As we got closer to May, we anticipated the end of intensive chemo. Bill's last CHOP treatment was in May and if all went according to plan, his CVC line would be removed on May 10 and he'd be free. But Bill was not looking good at all. The only thing that kept him out of a wheelchair was utter determination. His counts were low and he kept getting fevers pushing 100 degrees. Dr. Hagemeister's words about infections rang in my mind: likely to happen and likely to kill you.

It was April 29, 2004 and the kids had a program at school. As one of the teachers, I had been there since early in the morning and would stay until late in the night helping to clean up. We were having a silent auction and dinner following the program and several teachers remarked that Bill wasn't looking well. He didn't eat and he left with my mom and kids early. At 9:00 my phone rang. "My fever is 101," said Bill. We'd been told that 100.5 meant he needed to get to the emergency room. I left the school as my teacher friends hugged me and told me they would be praying. My friend Lynn wouldn't let me go alone. "I'll be fine," I told her, "I go down there all the time late at night." But Lynn wouldn't take no for an answer. She jumped into the passenger side of my SUV and called to tell her husband not to wait up for her. That's something for which I'll always be grateful. While we waited for the next several hours, I spent part of my time in the room with Bill but most of it out in the waiting area with Lynn. Bill was not speaking much. His skin was so very pale, it almost looked gray and all the light was gone from his eyes. I hated thinking it, but to me he looked like death. Out in the waiting area, Lynn and I had a Dr. Pepper and talked and even laughed a little. Her company was quite helpful in distracting me from fear.

Once the initial test results came back, the doctor told Bill he would have to be admitted to the hospital because his neutrophils were too low and he had a fever. By the time they admitted him it was 3:00 in the morning. I couldn't remember the last time I'd slept, but this day had been especially long. We had left in such a hurry that night that I hadn't checked to make sure Bill packed well. He hadn't. People with "chemo brain" should never try to pack a bag. All he had was pajama bottoms. As much as I wished I could stay by his side, I knew I'd have to go home to get his toothbrush and other essentials, so I kissed Bill goodbye and left with Lynn. It was good I wasn't alone driving back to The Woodlands.

When I arrived home, my mom woke up and hugged me. I took a warm bath and headed to bed for about two hours. Then I got the kids ready for school, comforting them about their dad and took my mom with me to the hospital. We stayed all day. My sister picked my children up from school and entertained them until I returned with my mom. Without saying anything, we all had the same fear. Was this the dreaded infection that would take his life? Even Bill seemed to have that fear.

Bill

I was lonely in that hospital room. I had trouble sleeping and I was a little scared. The room was nice. I was in the gynecology ward in a pretty room with posters about ovarian cancer. The hospital was full, and it was the only room available. I hadn't packed well and didn't have my sleeping pills, so the nursing staff brought me medicine to help me sleep at least a little.

During the night, I began to wonder if this infection was something serious enough to take my life. It wasn't the first time I had pictured Dana-Susan as a widow, but it seemed more real this time. I wasn't thinking too much about myself, but about the people I loved. I thought about my kids and how hard it would be for them to lose their daddy. I thought about my parents and what extreme pain it would cause them to lose another of their children to cancer. I decided that when I saw Dana-Susan again, I'd ask her to call them just in case this would be the last time they'd see me.

Dana-Susan

The next morning brought more violent weather. A tornado was in our town and another tornado was in a neighboring town. I couldn't get to the medical center. My in-laws would be driving down from Dallas that afternoon. I had planned on taking my sister with me to stay with Bill all day, but she and my mom were not budging on their decision to wait out the weather. All I could think was that my Bill was going to be alone. What if he takes his last breath all by himself? I couldn't stand it.

Finally, the weather calmed down and my sister and I left. We sat in the hospital room all day and when my in-laws arrived, I escorted them through the massive cancer center and to the hospital room where Bill lay barely awake. Later, we all (including Bill) took a little walk while we showed my mother and father-in-law the hospital. On the second floor is a beautiful historical look into the beginnings of this cancer center, built thanks to a foundation created by Monroe Anderson in the 1930s. Photos and videos showed the incredible advances made in cancer treatments over the years. My in-laws looked deeply troubled. "Why didn't they have all this when Michelle had leukemia," asked my mother-in-law.

Bill

Being in the hospital was unpleasant in many ways. I wanted to be at home in my own bed getting better there, but I was thankful for a place like MD Anderson where I could be kept alive when my body was trying to die. I felt sorry for my parents.

I knew it must be very painful for them to be there. I tried to pretend I was feeling better than I was so they wouldn't be afraid. I was glad Dana-Susan and her sister Anna were there for my mom and dad. They all left the hospital that evening together and suddenly I was in my room alone. I ordered dinner and hated it. I kept thinking about the fact that my wife, sister-in-law and parents were feasting at a seafood restaurant while I had this hospital food. I wanted to be with them. I wanted life and freedom from this disease. I longed to get up out of that bed and take my life back.

Dana-Susan

I spent the next couple of days alone with Bill in the hospital room and at home alone at night. My children had gone to stay with my brother. During the days, Bill mostly slept while I sat in his bed holding his hand. I hated leaving the hospital. My fear was that if he died, he would die alone.

But Bill didn't die. Dr. McLaughlin was the lymphoma doctor on call and I will never forget his walking into the room one Sunday morning and saying, "your counts are up and your fever is down, so we're sending you home." He added that they could go ahead and remove the CVC line from his arm since he was finished with intensive chemotherapy treatments. I wanted to kiss that man. That catheter had been a chain binding Bill to this disease. Its removal meant the end of chemo and the beginning of freedom. And here was a doctor saying we were removing it and my husband was going home to live.

Bill and I sat excitedly for the next couple of hours waiting for the nurse from Infusion Therapy to come and get that thing out of there. Suddenly we were happy. We were not so tired. When she came in, my mind was flooded with memories from months before when a 20-minute procedure to insert this thing had become three hours of torture. "This will come out easier than it went in won't it," asked Bill.

"Oh, it's easy," smiled the nurse. In less than five minutes we watched as she snipped and pulled and the long line that went from his wrist to his heart came out.

Bill was released that day. He was disconnected from his catheter, from his chemo, from his prison. Tears were forming in our eyes. Here was the moment we'd waited for. This was the time for dancing that jig. This marked the end of it. Peace flooded our hearts and minds. I kissed my survivor husband and we both felt truly blessed. We had been through this together and no one could take that from us. This was our moment to celebrate.

The ride back to The Woodlands was lovely. The skies were blue and the birds were singing. Bill was alive. That's all I could think about. My husband was not dead. He was alive. He had survived cancer and surely he would continue to survive it.

We couldn't wait for my mom to bring Morgan and Dylan home to us. They'd been having fun with their uncle, but had been quite distressed about their dad too. On their way home, they begged their grandma to take them to visit their daddy. She kept saying, "You'll have to wait and ask your mommy about that."

When they pulled into the driveway, I ran to greet them. They were nervously asking, "Where's Daddy, can we go see Daddy?" I only responded, "Well, I have a surprise for you." Then I walked down the hall and returned with their dad. They broke out into cheers.

"I have a surprise for you too," said Bill, hands behind his back. They waited in great expectation and when Bill pulled his arm out, they noticed immediately that his catheter was gone. "Now we can swim with you," they screamed. They'd waited for so long.

That was one great night. We didn't stay up late since we were all so exhausted, but we held each other and celebrated a great victory. We fought together as a family and this victory was ours. Healing would take a while and we all needed healing. But finally, we were on that road to achieving it.

A time to build up...

Bill

*B*efore being diagnosed with lymphoma, I had been regularly running three or four miles three times each week, swimming, and lifting weights. On my first visit with Dr. Hagemeister, he told me that my bones were too brittle to lift weights or run because the jarring impact could shatter them. I had extensive bone involvement with my disease. Swimming would be fine were it not for the CVC line in my arm which couldn't get wet. So I was left with walking and Pilates. But as I got farther into chemotherapy treatments, I got more and more tired. A lot of times, I would just lie on the couch staring at the clock.

Shadowbend Park was a pretty, tranquil park in The Woodlands with a sports field, a pool, a pond, and tennis courts. Often we'd pass by the park on Saturday mornings and see a banner there near water coolers. The sign read "The Leukemia & Lymphoma Society: Team In Training". "Is there some kind of race going on," Dana-Susan asked the first time we saw it. But then we continued seeing it every weekend. I was still finishing treatments, but Dana-Susan encouraged me to sometime stop by and see what this Team In Training was all about. I always had my reasons for not going. I was too sick. I was too tired. Why did I need to stop by anyway? I couldn't exactly join in if it was a race!

However, in May of 2004 those reasons dried up. I finished

chemotherapy and was released from the hospital. Coincidentally, I received a postcard in the mail inviting me to a Team In Training information meeting to be held at our local library. "You should go," Dana-Susan encouraged. My only excuse this time was that I didn't want to show up at this meeting as a bald-headed cancer patient. "It's the Leukemia Society," said Dana-Susan, "I think they can handle a bald-headed cancer patient."

On the morning of the meeting, I arrived about five minutes late. The meeting was in progress and someone directed me to an empty chair. As I took my seat, the lady leading the meeting began talking about training for marathons. Then a couple of coaches got up and started saying that before we knew it, we would be running more miles than we ever had before. The meeting went on with talk of fundraising. I was in the middle of the room and did not want to just get up and leave so I stayed and politely listened, but I knew I wasn't ready to start a big fundraising campaign or train for a marathon yet.

At the end of the meeting, I got up to talk to the young woman who led the meeting. Her name was Ally. I told her that I had just finished intensive chemo and that even though I had not run in more than six months, I might like to run with the group some. Having never had anyone who'd just completed aggressive chemo ask if they could run, she wasn't sure how to answer. She quickly introduced me to Coach Bill Dwyer. That would be the start of a beautiful friendship. I told Coach Bill I had just finished chemotherapy and would be continuing with less toxic cancer treatments for maybe another couple of years, but that I would like to train with his group if it was okay with him. He also had never been asked about this. Since I had two more years of treatments, he said he would like to have my doctor's permission. I knew that wouldn't be a problem.

I walked into that meeting that morning thinking this Team In Training could have been anything from a race event to a support group. When I left, I walked away with both – a training group and new support group – one that would help me get my life back.

With my doctor's permission, I began running with Team In Training (TNT). Soon I would learn that TNT is one of many fundraising campaigns at the Leukemia & Lymphoma Society. Dana-Susan and I both felt a little sad that we hadn't known about this organization when I was first diagnosed. They have all kinds of programs for families dealing with cancer from support groups to financial assistance. They have a program called First Connection in which cancer patients can talk to other patients who have a similar diagnosis and treatment plan and get some idea of what to expect. Through TNT, I would soon become even more involved with the Leukemia & Lymphoma Society.

Meanwhile, getting up early on Saturday mornings to run with TNT was building strength and endurance once again. Before cancer, swimming had been my true love and my longest distance to run had been four miles. Suddenly I was out there running long distances, even in the double digits. I wasn't as strong as I had been before cancer, but I could feel myself getting there and I was going to enjoy the journey.

Although I was still going to be doing rituximab treatments every three months and I was still pretty weak and pale, Coach Bill encouraged me to go ahead and pursue my dream of doing a triathlon. One was coming up at the beginning of October. It would be exactly five months after getting out of the hospital and finishing chemotherapy. And it would be the anniversary of my diagnosis with cancer. I wasn't sure I was up for such a big challenge.

Bill Dwyer is the kind of guy who makes you believe you can do anything. He's compassionate and genuine. His entire life he's been an athlete. In his high school days he was a wrestler from upstate New York. In the 1970's he moved to Houston and soon became a runner. He has run multiple marathons and ultra-marathons, including the Boston Marathon. But Coach Bill's passion for endurance sports is outweighed by his passion for people. Nothing brings him more pleasure than to see a new athlete cross the finish line in their first race and he'll cry tears of joy right along with them all.

When he suggested I do a triathlon so quickly, I was shocked. I wasn't exactly fit. I was still bearing the scars from chemo and my hair was nothing more than fuzz. But somehow, just because Bill said I could, I decided I would. Dana-Susan was all for it. She would support me in triathlon just as she supported me in cancer and life.

Getting back to swimming was one of the greatest joys of my life. I was nowhere near as fast as I'd once been, but just being in the pool was like a huge victory over cancer. Running was becoming more and more of a pleasure too. But the bike was fairly new to me. Dana-Susan, Morgan, Dylan and I had always ridden our bikes through the trails in town and I had been preparing to get into triathlon when I was diagnosed, but I had never been a cyclist. I had to learn a new sport and fast. It would not be easy, but after doing chemotherapy, I felt I could handle anything.

I was nervous, but filled with excitement as we left the hotel early that Sunday morning heading to the Stonebridge Ranch Triathlon in McKinney, Texas. We got there very early so I could check my bike and get body-marked. I needed a little extra time setting up my transition since this whole sport was new to me. It was a cold morning. I looked around at all the other triathletes there thinking how great it was to be a part of the world of fitness and sport once again. Less than five months earlier, I was in a hospital bed barely alive. But on this day, I was more than just alive. I was filled with energy and ready to go. I found Dana-Susan and the kids on the hill freezing. I kissed them as they wished me luck. Having them there was fitting. They'd all three been my biggest fans and support system through lymphoma. Now they were my biggest fans and support system in triathlon. Then I left them and lined up to start the race.

Dana-Susan

Since I'd never been to a triathlon, I wasn't sure where the best cheer spots were. Our friend Travis came out to cheer for Bill, so I just stuck with him. After we saw Bill exit the water and run to transition, we were excited. He looked happy and had a fairly fast swim, especially for someone who had just finished intensive chemotherapy.

I had no idea how long the bike would take. It was a sprint distance triathlon so the bike was 12.4 miles and not being too familiar with cycling, I couldn't even guess what his time would be. But soon, we saw him coming in on the bike and we all cheered loudly. Now he would only have five kilometers to run. We stood at the finish line awaiting him. My heart was beating quickly. It was hard to believe we were really here doing this. I'd seen him go from strong and athletic to sick and almost dead to strong and athletic once again.

When Bill came around the corner and over the hill towards the finish line that day, tears flowed down my cheeks. His smile was from ear to ear. His entire face glowed with great satisfaction. Morgan and Dylan cheered loudly and proudly. The three of us witnessed our hero defy a deadly disease and victoriously cross the finish line in that long-awaited triathlon. In that moment, on that unforgettable October morning, we experienced the thrill of victory like we never had before and we all felt like champions. We ran to him and I threw my arms around his neck and said, "I'm so proud of you." He glowed and grabbed the kids. On the way home I thought, "no matter what happens in life, nothing can take this day away from us."

With all the glory of that triathlon, it was hard to accept the reality that Bill had a disease that was completely incurable and that he had to continue treatments. For the next two years he would be continuing rituximab, the monoclonal antibody that kills the B cells. Every three months he would go in for an eight-hour treatment after lots of blood work and scans. So even though we felt like we'd won the war, the truth was the war raged on. Thankfully rituximab on its own did not have severe side effects. Bill's hair grew back, and he became stronger. We were thankful for a drug that could keep him in remission without making him sick. But two years of it were not easy. And having this lymphoma hovering over us was nerve-racking. Often, I found myself looking at his neck to see if I saw any tumors. Every time he itched or sweated, I wondered if it was cancer.

To make matters worse, I began to think we were all at risk. After all, we didn't know how Bill acquired this disease. Was it because of his dad's exposure to Agent Orange in Vietnam? Was it because I had been tested positive for Epstein Barr Virus? Did I give it to my kids? These questions ran through my mind on occasion, but I fought them and did my best to get on with life.

Fighting cancer is hard, exhausting work and we all fought it hard. We were tired and emotionally drained. It was time now to get up and get better.

A time to gain...

Dana-Susan

Whatever all we thought had been taken from us during cancer no longer mattered. We could choose to view this all as a terrible time of loss for our family. There was certainly much lost, but what we gained was far greater. The benefit resulting from the disease outweighed any feelings of loss. You could say we lost time, but we choose to believe we increased in time, time more precious. You could say we lost health. At the end of it all, though, we say we've never known greater health. We had always been active and healthy, but having endured the trauma of a deadly disease, we now had a deeper appreciation for our health. And we were not going to settle for just being physically fit anymore. With everything in our being, we had to get out there and prove to lymphoma that we had won, and it had lost. Triathlon is the sport that helped us prove our victory.

Bill

I began swimming competitively as a small boy. Although I participated in a variety of sports, swimming was always my favorite. In my early years I medaled most often in backstroke and then as I grew older, butterfly became my stroke. At the age of 23, I began volunteering as a swim coach for the Texas Amateur Athletic Federation. After work, I'd head straight to the pool. I loved coaching more than competing, but I continued to compete as well. Through the years I had many swimmers whom I'd say were amongst my favorites, but my most favorite was my wife. Dana-Susan was a great athlete with strong determination. She, too, had competed in many sports as a child and youth and had always been into physical fitness. When we got married, it was obvious we both belonged together on the swim team. She decided to get back into competition to spend more time with me and the other swimmers, most of whom were teenagers and adults in their twenties. We created some of our best memories in those couple of years. We hosted pasta parties and special events for the team and traveled every weekend through the summer months.

After we moved to The Woodlands, I volunteered there too, coaching a youth swim league. Dana-Susan and I were no longer competing because by then we had two kids, but we continued swimming and participated in a variety of physical activities.

One summer afternoon, we sat with our friends Debra and Gregg. We'd been swimming laps and the subject of triathlon came up. Debra had been doing triathlons and thought we might want to race in one. I was more than a little interested, but I could tell Dana-Susan was not at all. She said her days of competition were over and she was meant to be a mom now. For me, the idea of branching out into this new, exciting sport seemed perfect.

I had already been running a couple of days a week, swimming almost daily, and lifting weights. The only thing I needed was to learn more about cycling. It was decided. I would train for a triathlon.

Only a few weeks later, I was diagnosed with cancer and it seemed like that dream was lost forever. Somehow, even in the darkest moments, when my body was drained of energy and almost lifeless, the hope of doing that triathlon remained alive in me. Sometimes I think it was what drove me to fight extra hard. I couldn't die without doing that tri.

When I finally finished chemo and Coach Bill encouraged me to register for the triathlon in McKinney, I felt alive again. I didn't have much time to train, but I put forth my greatest effort. Triathlon was my way of getting in cancer's face and saying, "You lose!"

Dana-Susan

After seeing Bill cross the finish line in McKinney, I was motivated. I decided I needed to compete in a triathlon of my own. Two were coming up, one in our hometown and one in Austin. I chose the Capital of Texas Triathlon in Austin to be my first. The only bike I owned was a mountain bike and since I thought the only triathlon I'd ever do was this one, I decided to borrow a bike instead of buying one. I coached myself on the bike which later I'd learn wasn't too wise. Since I'd already been a competitive swimmer, I didn't seek help with that either and the run, well, it was just as natural as it had been when I was a child. I actually learned through training that I loved running. My first triathlon would be a sprint distance which consisted of a 750-meter swim, a 12.4-mile bike and a 5-kilometer run. That same day, Bill would compete in his first Olympic distance, a

1500-meter swim, a 24.8-mile bike and a 10-kilometer run. His event began before mine and he finished in time to see me cross the finish line. Hearing him cheer for me was one great moment. We hugged and talked non-stop on the way home about how much fun we'd had. Again, we felt strong. We were getting our lives back and I had a feeling we'd get them back better than before.

There is such camaraderie with Team In Training participants all over the country. When you're racing in an event and you hear someone scream "Go Team" it really gets you pumped. TNT began in 1988 when a man named Bruce Cleland decided to run the New York City Marathon to raise money in support of leukemia research because his daughter was battling the disease. Bruce and other participants raised $320,000 in that first run and since then Team In Training has raised more than $1.5 billion dollars for research into cures for blood cancers. Participants sign on to compete in a triathlon, marathon, century bike ride or other endurance sport while raising a designated amount in order to participate. They receive professional coaching and various clinics on nutrition, hydration, stretching and other sports-related topics. They are assigned an "honored teammate", a person who has battled out blood cancer, for whom to race. Bill was happy to become an honored teammate for our training area. We viewed this as both an honor and a duty. Our job was to make people aware of the effect lymphoma has on families and to thank them for joining the war against cancer.

Our family will always feel a huge depth of gratitude to Coach Bill Dwyer who encouraged us to join the team long before we knew we were ready. It was on our own initiative that we attended the first meetings, but because of Coach Bill we continued to pursue goals in endurance sports we never dreamed of.

After getting my first taste of triathlon, I bought my own bike and continued to compete. More and more I found I enjoyed the run so one night it hit me: I'll do a marathon. In an instant, I made the decision to become a fundraising participant for Team In Training and run the Houston Marathon. Within 10 minutes I'd already written a fundraising letter and made a plan and the season hadn't even begun. The next night, I received a phone call from a good friend, Angie Rizzo. She had received a TNT postcard in the mail and wanted to join and do the Houston Marathon. I told her we would be on the same team and we were both excited.

The kick-off party for the winter marathon season was in early August. Bill was asked to be the main speaker for all six training locations that would be in attendance. He asked me to join him and speak too. He thought people needed to see me and the kids on the stage and truly be aware that cancer doesn't just affect the patient, but the entire family. It was a true honor to get up there and tell the audience how much we appreciated what they were doing. They were heroes in our eyes, there to raise money for diseases many of them had never intimately experienced. Bill and I spoke as our children stood holding our hands and I felt truly thrilled to kick off a new season and train for my first marathon. I also realized the simple act of being willing to tell our story was going to go a long way in bringing healing to us and many others.

When I sent out my fundraising letter, I sent it with a second page attached explaining who I was running my race for. It struck me that I needed to run my race to honor God for giving me the body, heart, and mind to do this race. And I also needed to run in honor of 26 people who were heroes in the war against blood cancers. I dedicated each of my 26 miles to a hero, some of whom had fought cancer and won and others who had become casualties in the war against cancer. I ran in memory of our friend Chad and my sister-in-law I never got to meet. I ran for our friend Robert who lost his life to lymphoma while I was in training. I ran for Dr. Hagemeister's mom, Selma, who was at the time, a 90-year-old survivor of lymphoma and a fighting champion just like her son. I ran for my brother, Luke Park, and I ran in special honor of my husband Bill, who never ceases to amaze me. Knowing I was running for all those people made this race all that more important. I was raising money and committing myself to all these people and I couldn't let anyone down.

Bill was registered to run the marathon too and it would be his first. But he was also training for his longest distance yet in triathlon. In October, right after he and I competed once again in the McKinney triathlon celebrating the second anniversary of his diagnosis, Bill would compete in a half iron distance triathlon in Montgomery, Texas. This race consisted of a 1.2-mile swim, a 59-mile bike and a 13.1-mile run. It was a super hilly course, and I was thrilled to see him thoroughly enjoying his training. He continued to do his rituximab treatments, having one in August and would have his next one following the triathlon in November.

I missed his race because of a prior commitment, but Coach Bill phoned me as he finished each leg of the race and finally finished in an incredible six hours and 14 minutes. It was unbelievable. He was still doing cancer treatments, but was able to finish a half iron distance triathlon in six hours! When he got home, he was on a high like I hadn't seen in a long time. Finally I was beginning to believe we were in a time of peace.

One week later, while out at the lake, I saw a lump on Bill's chest. It felt like the world suddenly stopped. "What's that," I asked, frightened. Bill had not noticed it before. It wasn't small. I begged him to call his doctor, but he said it was pointless since his appointment was so soon. But as days passed and Bill was just as frightened, he decided to send his doctor an email. His doctor said he definitely needed to see it right away.

Bill

It was hard to believe this disease might be back. I'd seen so much triumph in these past several months. How could I have this thing on my chest? I tried at first to make light of it, but I was truly afraid. Dana-Susan wasn't holding back her thoughts and fears either. She was training so hard for her marathon and dealing with the recent loss of her grandfather. Now her husband has a large lump on his chest. My mind began to race with the idea of going through chemo again. Then it hit me that chemo might not be an option now. What if I needed a stem cell transplant? This was tough to bear. Each day I tried to remain positive, but this bump on my chest wasn't getting any smaller.

Dana-Susan

Those few weeks had been quite harsh. Our friend Robert died after a five year battle against lymphoma. The next day, my grandfather died. I injured myself in training. And Bill had a lump. Where did all that lovely peace go?

Amye, a beautiful physician's assistant entered the exam room first and looked at the lump. She thought they might need to biopsy it. Then Dr. Hagemeister came in and looked at it. He showed us on his computer what this lump looked like inside. In his very professional opinion, it was "weird". He did not believe it to be malignant although more tests would be done to determine that for sure. He thought it was a damaged muscle. I nearly laughed out loud. Imagine that! When all this began two years ago, Bill thought that lump in his armpit was a damaged muscle and it turned out to be cancer. Now here we were thinking this lump on his chest was cancer and it might just turn out to be a damaged muscle. After some tests, we discovered Dr. Hagemeister was right. It was just a damaged muscle.

Having to take three weeks off of training because of my injury, I was not pleased. But I listened to my doctor and only swam laps for those few weeks. When my ankle was healed, I resumed training. It was a huge commitment. Finding time to put in my runs was not easy with my busy schedule.

When January rolled around, I had raised almost $13,000 and was tapering for the race. It was incredible. As Bill and I awaited our first marathon, we felt even more alive. It had been a tough training season with death and injury and fear, but it had also been one of the greatest experiences of our lives.

On January 15, 2006, I crossed the finish line in the Houston Marathon. Seven minutes later, Bill finished. It had been a perfect day. And to my surprise (since I never wear a watch and had no idea of my pace) I qualified to run the Boston Marathon. Three months later, Bill and I made a quick trip to Boston and I had another of the greatest times of my life.

Through the two years of rituximab treatments, Bill remained free of cancer, and we continued with life. We returned to our many loves and found many new ones. Our kids returned to their sports. They both thrived at swimming and being a part of the Hurricanes swim team was like being part of a family. The kids also began to compete in triathlon events. Dylan was only four years old when he did his first. It was wonderful. Cancer had been a family affair, so now our sports became the same.

Bill

Being out there competing and watching my wife and children

compete was more of a triumph than I could have ever imagined. It made my quarterly trips to have a treatment not seem so bad. I knew they'd eventually come to an end, and I had a good feeling that things would only get better for me physically.

Sometimes I had concerns about the effect of all these drugs. I wondered how deep the damage was from chemo and if the constant killing of my B cells was going to produce negative results eventually. Often, I found myself suffering from cold-like symptoms and found running pretty tough on my body. Every time I went in for a treatment, I felt just slightly nervous about the results of my scans. Mostly I felt confident that no cancer would be found, but I was realistic enough to know that I was still fighting a deadly disease. With each visit, I grew more and more confident and more and more excited about finishing. My scheduled date to finish treatments was June 2006. My doctor had decided that two years of maintenance treatments was enough and he was honest when he told me he didn't know for sure how my body would react to continuing to kill my good, healthy B cells.

Dana-Susan got busy planning an "End of Treatment" party for me. There were many good friends with whom we wanted to celebrate. They had stood against cancer with us and they deserved a time of celebration with us. As we walked into the lymphoma clinic for that visit before my final treatment, we both felt eager to get it done. But we felt a little sentimental too. This place was a home to us. The doctor, the nurse and physician's assistant, even the scheduler, had become part of our "family". In some ways, we almost felt a little sad that it was over. This chapter in our lives had been long and had impacted us so greatly, it was hard to let it go and enter the new chapter.

That appointment with Dr. Hagemeister was pleasant. We talked to him about the usual topics – triathlon, fitness, everything but lymphoma. And as we walked away from the clinic that evening, we felt a happy calmness. We spent the night in the hotel across the street from the medical center. We had to be back for the treatment early in the morning. It amused us that another storm blew through town. Again, thunder and lightning and the threat of hurricane-like conditions reminded us of the first treatment in this place 2 ½ years before. Again, I was scheduled in the same Ambulatory Treatment Center. We sat in the same seats we'd sat in 2 ½ years ago and reminisced. Then, we'd been afraid. Now, we were satisfied. Then we were entering the dark unknown. Now we were leaving it behind.

After several hours of infusion, the nurse came in to give me my final drip to clean me out. Then I was disconnected, bandaged and discharged. We grabbed our computer and movies. We looked around the room to make sure we had all our things. We looked at each other with contentment and left. It was finished.

The celebration with friends was perfect. We had great food and played fun games. We celebrated the success of surviving cancer with our friends. It was done. Now we could move on and conquer new things. Morgan, Dylan, Dana-Susan and I had been through it all together as a team. We were winners.

A time to speak...

Dana-Susan

Fighting for Bill's life was the greatest challenge we'd known as a family. It brought us closer together in the end, but defending ourselves against this giant of an enemy was not easy. It came after us quick and hard and nearly beat us. Afterward, we decided it was time to pick up a sword and go on the offense in the war against cancer.

Our "sword" was our story. We used our voices to raise funds and awareness by sharing our story with people wherever we went and by encouraging others who'd been battling cancer to do the same. We volunteered a great deal of our time with our local chapter of the Leukemia & Lymphoma Society. I volunteered some at MD Anderson. We traveled and spoke at various Team In Training functions. We spoke to members of congress about funding for cancer research. We spoke on television and the radio and wrote articles for magazines and newspapers. Bill and I and even our children learned to use our voices to speak on behalf of those who were continuing to fight for their lives because we felt it was our duty. We couldn't think of a better cause for our family. Our lives have been deeply affected by cancer. We've lost family and friends to these diseases and we almost lost Bill. It was time to get out there and do something.

Our children's suffering turned to something positive when their story was published. When Bill was sick, I began to write down the many precious things Morgan and Dylan were saying and doing. When we talked about their dad's disease and our family's duty to fight it, I found their words inspiring and beautiful. I put their words and illustrations into book form and gave it to Bill as a Father's Day gift after he'd gone into remission. He appreciated it and began to share it with others who asked for copies. I continued making copies until finally I realized we needed to give it away so it could help kids who were dealing with a parent's cancer diagnosis.

One of our other favorite people is a lovely lady named Cherry Evans. She was the Patient Services Manager for the Texas Gulf Coast Chapter of the Leukemia & Lymphoma Society. Cherry felt certain that this book would touch people's hearts and benefit those with young children as they might find it helpful in explaining the complexities of cancer. With our permission, she printed copies for people. Eventually, their book "Our Daddy's Cancer: How We Helped Him Fight" was published in hopes that many more lives would be impacted. Our kids were touching lives simply by being brave little soldiers in the war against cancer.

We all do our parts to continue to wage war against lymphoma and other cancers. It had originally come against us and we'd been the victims. Now it was our turn to go against it. The greatest part of it was that we were not alone. Many millions of patients and family members and friends and doctors and nurses and volunteers and heroic people all over the world fight every day. What an honor for us to be a part of this vast community of brave souls all around the world.

Not a day goes by that we feel regret for the difficulty we knew during cancer. Never are we sad or bitter that this ugly tormenter blew through our home like a great storm. No, we feel honored- honored to have been chosen to fight this good fight, honored to have kept the faith in the most heated of battles, honored to have met some of the most amazing people we've ever known. I'm glad God saw fit to give us this opportunity. Seeing my husband stand up to cancer and fight it back was amazing. My admiration for him shall never cease. And being right by his side during the most horrible times of our lives was a blessing. How privileged was I that I got to be the one holding his hand before he endured bone marrow tests or lying in bed with him as toxic chemicals pumped into his body. I was the one driving him to and from the medical center. I was the one up with him at night when he vomited. I was the one taking his temperature, cleaning and dressing his catheter and giving him daily care like a nurse. From the depths of my soul, I have loved my husband in his sickness and in his health, in the good times and bad, and I will love him 'til death parts us.

Bill

Fighting for my life was a privilege for which I'll always be grateful. I learned that surviving cancer requires courage not only from the patient, but from his family and friends as well. Without a team of warriors helping me battle this disease, I know I wouldn't have survived, but the truth remains that the main fight, the depth of warfare, belongs to the patient. The disease attacked my body, and it was up to me to decide to declare war against it. Some of the ways I actively fought lymphoma were by getting up and trying to live as normal a life as possible. I refused to let cancer rob me of my joy. And I decided not to complain or feel sorry for myself. I didn't want to play the victim.

Having lymphoma was in some ways the worst thing that I ever experienced. But ultimately, it was one of the greatest blessings of my life. Having suffered it, I am part of that club of survivors, and I'm honored to be part. But the truth is, courageous people fight their diseases every day and do not survive. Courage doesn't save your life. Ultimately, we need more funding for research so that more brave souls can win their battles against cancer. Our family is dedicated to this cause.

My hope is that our story will inspire people to wage war against their diseases and troubles no matter what they are. If that doesn't happen, then we fought in vain.

"I have fought the good fight, I have finished the race, I have kept the faith." (1 Timothy 4:7)

This story was originally published in 2007 and distributed at educational conferences to help patients and caregivers through a cancer diagnosis. Since then, the Crews family has continued to keep their promise to "go on the offense in the war against cancer". In April 2008, Bill and Dana-Susan crossed the finish line at the Ford Ironman Arizona in Tempe, proving once again that cancer lost its attack on them. Following this race, they formed a nonprofit organization called Remission Run, Inc. whose signature event was the Bill Crews Remission Run. This event and organization was used to raise funds for the Lymphoma Tissue Bank at MD Anderson Cancer Center. The Crews family has also continued to raise awareness and funding through the Leukemia & Lymphoma Society, the Lymphoma Research Foundation, and other local cancer organizations.

As of December 2021, Bill and Dana-Susan live in Fort Worth, Texas. Morgan is a teacher in the Dallas area and Dylan is finishing his senior year at Texas A&M University where he is an engineering major. Each of the four of them has participated in fundraising for cancer research individually and as a team. Through the various organizations they have worked with, they have helped raise millions of dollars to develop better therapies for cancer patients. They are not finished yet.

You can read more and find helpful cancer resources by visiting www.bellasteri.com/resources.

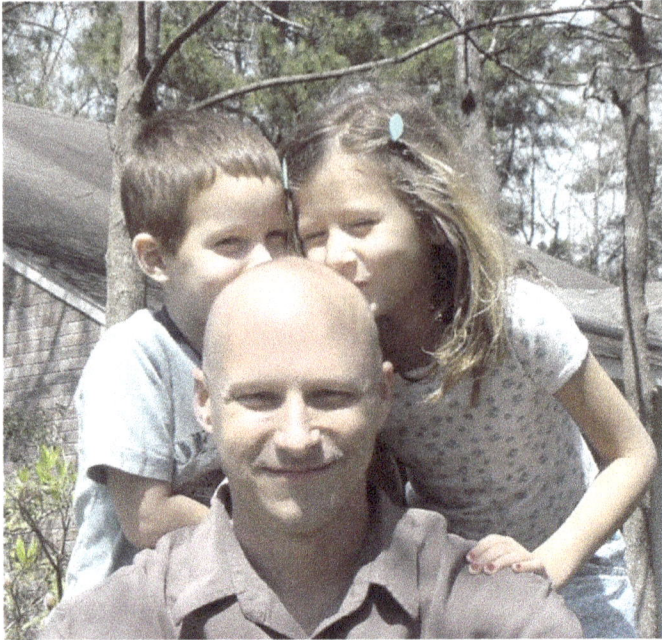

"Bald Kisses"

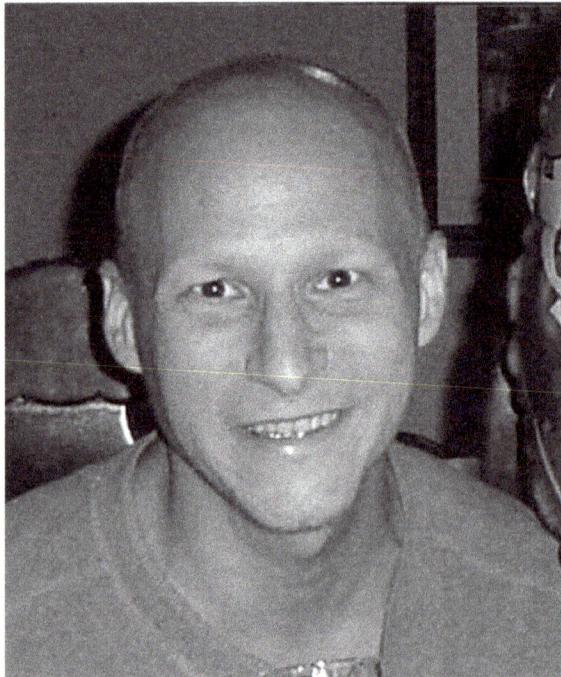

Bill smiling after being released from the hospital in May 2004

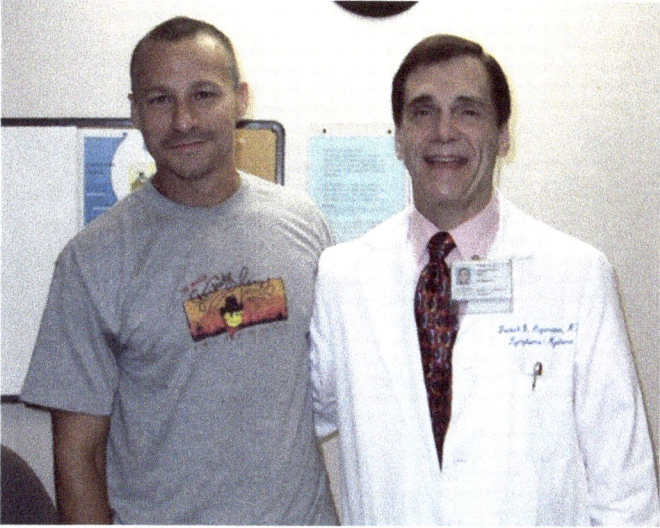

Bill Crews with Dr. Fredrick Hagemeister at MD Anderson Cancer Center

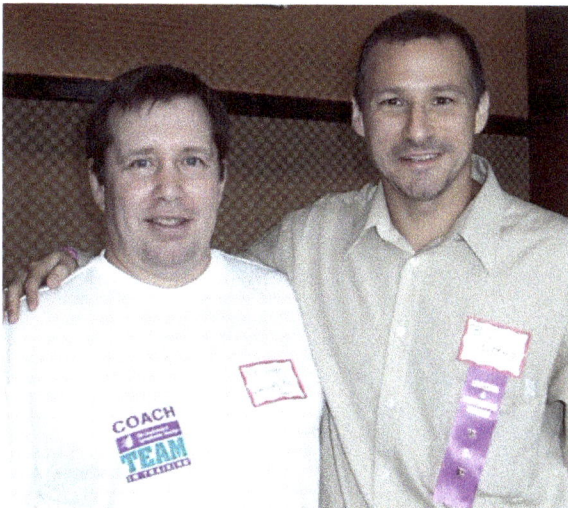

Bill Crews with Coach Bill Dwyer at a Team In Training event in Houston, Texas

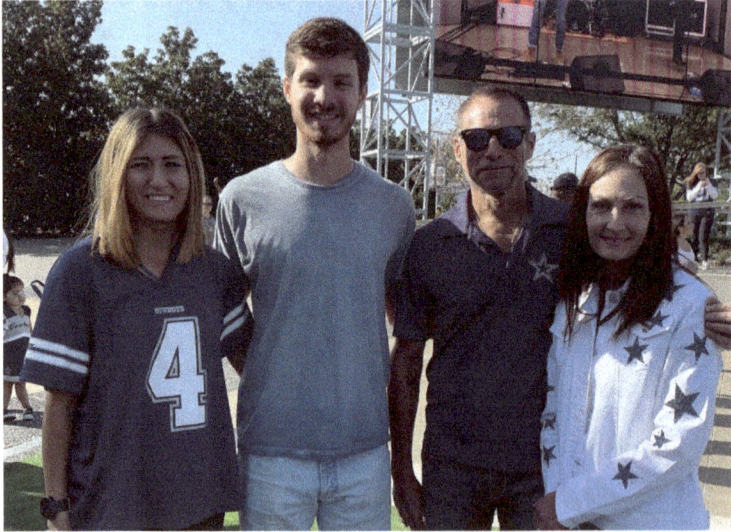

The Crews Family in 2021: Morgan, Dylan, Bill and Dana-Susan